DYING TO LIVE:
A REBEL'S JOURNEY
OUT OF THE ABYSS

*A Minister's Personal Journey
of Trials and Triumphs*

Rev. Betty R. Jones, Ph.D.

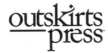

outskirts
press

Outskirts Press, Inc.
http://www.outskirtspress.com

ISBN: 978-1-4787-9692-3

Cover illustration by Kestrel Erickson

Outskirts Press and the "OP" logo are trademarks belonging to Outskirts Press, Inc.

PRINTED IN THE UNITED STATES OF AMERICA

TABLE OF CONTENTS

Part II

ACKNOWLEDGEMENTS

Writing this book was the hardest thing I have ever done. And without my family and the support of unwavering friends, I doubt that I would have ever written my memoirs. Throughout the years I started and stopped writing. Grief sometimes overtook me, and many rough drafts were thrown away. But, as years passed, I knew that I owed it to my grandchildren to tell the "real" story of our losses no matter how painful it may have been for me.

Admittedly, writing the manuscript became much easier when I could openly acknowledge that the deaths of my three children could cause mental depression. I acknowledge stigma as a culprit as it relates to mental health in the African American community. And to this end, I acknowledge both the Interdenominational Theological Center and Southern Regional Hospital's Pastoral Care departments. The verbatims and directives were priceless.

On the pages of "Dying to Live: A Rebels Journey out of the Abyss" I have tried to tell my grandchildren the heartbreaking story that is our story: Thank you Gerald, Ryan, Nasyir and Atya for accepting my desire not to talk about your parents and the causes of their deaths until now. You have been real troupers! Thank you, family members and friends, who repeatedly encouraged me to write a book, yet respected my desire not to write or talk about the pain-filled events. I recognize and acknowledge each one of you for respecting my privacy.

I also wish to acknowledge Deni Sinteral-Scott of Outskirts Press for her patience as I slowed the process at various intervals because I needed time to regroup. I also acknowledge Outskirts Press' editor for great editorial work.

Further, I wish to acknowledge the great work of Kestrel Erickson for the book cover. You are a very talented artist and I appreciate your perseverance in attaining the goal that I sought.

Last, but not least, I acknowledge two churches from the North Georgia United Methodist Conference: Bright Star United Methodist & County Line United Methodist for the many ways that you allowed me to work through my pain. You are both thoughtful and unique in your own way, and I thank you both.

FOREWORD

During my career as a professor in theological and religious studies, I frequently encountered gifted, talented, motivated and faith-filled students enrolled in seminary and theological school preparing to serve in churches, denominations and non-traditional ministries. From the first time I met Betty Jones, I knew that she would make a significant contribution to Christian ministry. In addition to possessing all the qualities identified above, her stylish dress, strong preaching voice and effervescent smile set her apart. It was only years later as we participated in a mission study travel seminar I facilitated to Kenya and Tanzania, while sitting in a van at the Zanzibar open market, that she shared with me her story of the death and loss of her three children and her husband. Hers is truly an amazing story, and I am glad that she not only has pursued doctoral degrees that have enabled her to further study academically critical issues related to the intersection of trauma, faith and mental health, but that she has also written this book, Dying to Live: A Rebels Journey Out of the Abyss.

While the book does many things, one of the most important is to call attention to our spirituality, that quality of being concerned with the human spirit, or soul, as opposed to material or physical things. Dr. Jones memoir encourages us to examine these current days in which we are living and to see in them an opportunity to embrace a deeper sense of spirituality.

As we attend to Dr. Jones' narrative, we can better understand how the human spirit is viewed as the real core of a person's being, and how it includes our intellect, emotions, reasoning, memories, perceptions and other mental abilities. As you read Dying to Live, you begin to see in this one life story how traumatic events cause us to experience pain, loss, and discomfort, and how such trauma also can actually help us ask important questions, to choose life, and make good decisions to move forward in hope. Yes, death, loss and change are an ordinary part of life, but when we are caught up in rapid change, our moral and ethical compass can place us on shaky ground.

What I like most about the book is how Dr. Jones poignantly and meaningfully describes her personal journey: the good, the bad and the ugly. She chooses her own path to faithfulness without knowing the outcome, and by doing so she invites us to embrace our own spirituality, our true, identity and to choose self-care and mental wellness. To men and women who may feel broken and dis-spirited, this book teaches that within each of us is the capacity to connect to a more meaningful life. For those who currently are at a good place in life mentally and spiritually, it is a reminder to take time to look, listen and really see those around us, and to offer a sense of community and hope.

More importantly, Dying to Live is an important reminder that there is much in life and in our American culture that can damage our human capacity to connect with others at the level of compassion and shared personal experiences. Yet, during her personal journey of trials and triumphs, Dr. Jones allow us to see how by connecting to her grandchildren through love and compassion that she overcame the damage and disruption that death and the loss loved ones did to her spirit. She reminds us that because we are spiritual human beings, and though traumatic situations in life may cause us to become dis-spirited, our spirit can be restored, renewed, and refreshed.

M. Snulligan Haney
Rev. Marsha Snulligan Haney, PhD

- Retired Professor of Missiology and Religions of the World, Interdenominational Theological Center, Atlanta, Georgia

- Honorably Retired Clergy, Presbyterian Church, USA

PART I

JONES

THE TWO OF us were alone when out of the blue she said, "Mommy, I am just tired, I can't take it anymore!" I was taken aback but I said, "Baby, if you are tired, just go to sleep. If you're worried about the boys, you don't have to worry; we will take good care of them!"

Two weeks later, and 16 and 1/2 months after she became ill, she said, "goodnight" for the final time. She said goodnight to feeding tubes, hospital rooms, surgeries, and pain and suffering.

Death is ugly, it is evil, and it can send the strongest person spiraling out of control. I stayed in the eye of "Storm Death" for five long years. But it was my rebellious nature that helped me withstand the brutal beatings of relentless storms. My rebellious nature refused to accept the status quo. My rebellious nature gave me the impetus to question God. My rebellious nature helped me fight back from the abyss. I am a "rebel with a cause." But I hasten to add that, although rebels may have a cause and may even be crafty and may think outside the box, death does not always allow room for thinking, because death comes like a thief in the night. But rebels are crafted differently and often look at death as a challenge to overcome. However, a rebel's journey into the darkness of death is not a challenge that must be won. Death may have us suspended in the abyss--a dark and dreary place--but rebels view it as a temporary holding place while God crafts them for purposeful living. Uncanny as it may seem, a rebel knows that with every struggle and every attempted takeover of their existence, God has already devised a plan of escape. Perhaps this is the reason rebels consistently defy the odds. They understand that it is up to them to figure out God's plan. For certain, rebels do not roll over on the tracks of life and wait for the train to roll over them, even though death may be imminent. Their minds shift into gear and they immediately think of ways to get off the tracks. Rebels think of a way out of the abyss. Rebels think of ways to live.

When death claimed my only daughter, I was thrown off balance and began to slip into the unknown where I found myself gasping for air. In the midst of my gasping, I heard a familiar voice urging me to remember where I came from, reminding me that a merciful God was still available to me. I was a "rebel" with a cause. The spirit of rebellion that existed in my mother was exemplified throughout my rebellious life. This voice was not new to me. I'd heard it many times before. My mother was her usual self. She said, "Don't you dare give up. Ask God to have mercy on you."

My mother knew the power and might of a true and living God. She taught me by example and the lessons I learned were evident throughout a very tumultuous five year journey into the abyss. I thank God for my mother and the things of God that she taught me. She taught me about God's grace and mercy and I know without a doubt that it was God's grace and mercy that sustained me throughout this terrifying journey.

The journey into the abyss was hellacious. Every time I thought about returning to some sense of normalcy, all hell broke loose. Thankfully, rebels are born. By God's grace they are born to survive the perils of life and there may be many. The storms in their lives are relentless. They just keep on coming. Perhaps in their creation God places a special anointing on them as they are being prepared and continuously crafted by God. I am not a rabble-rouser, but I have always had a spirit of rebellion deep down inside of me. I attribute that spirit to my mother. I was born to be a rebel. It was ingrained in me as a little girl. I saw it in her. I witnessed it in how my mother operated in her spiritual life, in her business life, and in her personal life. Frances always had a way of handling things in unusual ways. She loved God and she loved the church but she did not allow the church to dictate how she should live. She gave of herself and her sustenance willingly to the church but she maintained a hands-off approach to church folk who tried to penetrate her business life or personal life. I recall hearing that she had once been referred to in a community newspaper (did not call her by name but said just enough). What did they want to do that for? Frances was no joke! From what I hear, Frances shut down the entire publication. She did not bite her tongue in business matters, or in "matters of the heart." Talk about rebellion, Frances was married four times. She was a lovely well-put-together woman. She may have been lovely, but I saw the "rebel' in her rise up on many occasions with those who thought they had a "free ride." Not with Frances.

And by God's grace, Frances raised a rebellious daughter. I observed a first-class rebel who always went against the grain. I knew that it was in my blood to be just like her. Just as I knew that I was born to be a rebel, I also knew that there was an unexplainable force holding the reins as I spiraled into the abyss. God was holding the reins because God knew beforehand that He could not let me go. It is this undeniable God thing that some rebels have within that makes them who they are. Rebels have to arrive at their own truths. It does not mean that rebels are not human or have supernatural powers. They do not; it simply means that they are fighters. It also means that they will take action when others will not. Rebels stand up for what they believe in.

Even though a part of me died after the death of my beloved Valarie; and even though her death had me descending into the abyss, I knew that I could not let go of God. As I descended, I heard Frances speaking firmly, encouraging me to hold on and don't let go. She said, "Stay there, you will be alright."

But my rebellious spirit would not let me stay there lifelessly in suspension. At the time, I still had a husband, two sons, and four grandchildren to live for, and I also knew that God was not through with me yet. I was hanging by a thread while suspended but I was hanging on.

And just when I thought that I was on my way back from the depths of hell, my youngest son died. The shock of his death was more than any mother should have to endure, and the struggle to find my way back was the hardest thing I have ever had to do. But a merciful God held me close and He wouldn't let go. God held me in suspension while I fought my way out of hell.

Losing my darling baby boy sent me into an unimaginable tailspin and I had to fight with every fiber of my being to keep my sanity. And fight I did because I knew deep down inside that letting go would be too easy. I had to pray like I had never prayed before. I wanted to dance with my baby boy again. The last dance at his wedding couldn't possibly be the end.

There is something intriguing about me and dancing. I would never win a dancing competition, but I have always loved to dance. Just as I danced with Ryan when Valarie was dying, I danced with William (aka Billy) at his wedding two months prior to his disappearance and ultimate death. Fourteen months after Billy died, my oldest son Charles and the last of my three children died and I had danced with him at a family member's wedding. What I would give if I could have one last dance with my sons again! But it was not to be.

Rebels take a different approach to most situations and will sometimes plead their case to God and anyone who will listen. Pleading with Charles did not help. Pleading with God did not help. Reminding God and Charles that he was all that I had left did not help. The night that the call came about his death, I knew instinctively that it was about Charles. The belief that I had in my psychotic state was that Charles died because I had tried to bargain with God. Foolish me; I knew better. God cannot be bargained with.

Foolish or not, I tried everything, because my life was crumbling right in front of my eyes. I was in the fight of my life. Losing a child is the most devastating thing that can happen to a parent; imagine losing three. As parents we never expect our children to die before we do. Our expectation is that our children will be around to help take care of us when we grow older and cannot take care of ourselves. This is an interesting phenomenon because my daughter was deeply concerned about me. She always said that she wanted to be around to take care of me when I grew old. Now she is gone, and although I have four loving grandchildren, only one of them has remained in close proximity to where I live and he is constantly looking for other areas to live. As the years go by, I wonder who will see to it that I am cared for.

As I ponder who will take care of me when I am no longer able to take care of myself, I am reminded that I'm not a "rebel without a cause." God has always provided a cause and I have not had to look very far. My causes have always been "in your face." God has kept me pretty busy over my adult life, but I won't complain. I won't complain because no matter what "cause" God has given me, God has always provided what I needed to take action. And just as God has provided what I needed to take action when my causes where "in your face," God has already provided what I need to take care of me when I can no longer take care of myself. For instance, God already knows what tomorrow will bring just as He knew that I slept with a pillow over my face by day because I could not sleep at night after Charles' death. God also knew that the day would come when I'd begin to fight back. When the time came I had to take the pillow from my face, throw it on the floor, get up off the couch, and be about the business of caring for my family. That is what rebels do! They do not accept the status quo for anything. God knew that when the time was right I would shake off the grip of death and handle my responsibilities. But until then, I would stay suspended in the abyss like a zombie; unable to experience the beauty of life and wondering why God had not taken me instead of my children. But finally God gave me the "courage to be" whole again. It took me a while to come to a place of acceptance of God's plan but when I did, the pillows flew off of my face and I faced the fact that if God had wanted me He would have taken me instead of the children.

I did not see it coming because God does not show us everything. He does not have to. But seven years after Charles' death, I was dealt another blow. Basil, my beloved husband, died from pancreatic cancer. With the exception of Valarie, God in His infinite wisdom had protected me from the ordeal of watching those close to me die. But Basil died within two months of learning that he was in the fourth stages of cancer. He stayed in the hospital for one month after the diagnosis. And God gave me strength once again. I had to put on my running shoes so that I could run between the hospital every day, run to my neighbor's or school to pick up my grandchildren, get their dinner, see that they were doing their homework, and work on my Doctor of Ministry degree. I am amazed that I could remain standing. But wait, it wasn't me; it was that undeniable rein that held me when I could not hold myself. It had to be Jesus! When Basil finally came home, I wanted to give up on school and stay at home to care for him but he insisted on my staying in school. I kept going to school even though my professors advised me to take a semester off. Staying in seminary during this devastating crisis in my life helped me keep my sanity. Besides, rebels don't quit; they are expected to defy expectations.

As it were, Basil's journey to the beyond had taken some strange twists and turns prior to his bout with cancer. He lived another twelve years after Valarie's death, and another seven years after

Charles' death even though he had to have emergency open heart surgery five months after Charles passed away. In fact, he nearly died on the operating table and had to be resuscitated three times before the doctors could stabilize him. I thank God that the doctors kept working on him. It would have been too much if they had let him just slip away. Basil was my rock! He took care of the boys while I lingered in the abyss.

I was in a place where I did not try to be present for quite some time. Ryan was thirteen when Basil finally died and it was very hard for him to lose his grandfather. As for Gerald, he had always clung to me. I had just about given up the desire to come back from the abyss after his mother and uncles died. But one day I saw his face as he crept quietly around the room in an attempt not to disturb me. The perplexed look on his face asked the question: "Are you going to leave me too?" That look gave me the will and impetus to begin fighting my way back. I began to beg God to help me sleep at night so that I could take care of my grandsons. The look on Gerald's face broke my heart. After all, God had placed the boys in our care and they had to be my primary concern. The proudness of a rebel rose up in me ferociously and I knew that I had to fight harder to get back so that I could take care of my beloved grandsons. I began talking to myself and I had to keep telling myself: "If God wanted me, God would have taken me.' If God wanted me, God would have taken me. Stop trying to take over God's work.' Do what you were crafted to do."

I had to get a grip on the depression that was pulling me into the abyss. As it were, the boys had not been told that their dearly beloved uncles had died. My eldest grandson began to ask why neither of his uncles had been to Georgia to visit. Finally, I concocted a story about both being sick and unable to travel. I knew eventually I would have to tell Gerald the truth. I had already cried out to God at Charles' graveside, "How am I supposed to tell the boys about their uncles' deaths?" One of my friends looked at me and said, "God will give you the strength." I had already refrained from telling them about their Uncle Billy. But God gave me the strength one day to tell Gerald that they were dead. He looked at me all wide-eyed and said, "No way!" Telling him the truth about his uncles was the hardest thing I have ever had to do. I am thankful that Ryan was too young to ask questions. His life was wrapped up in his immediate family. And God was merciful because after I told Gerald about his uncles, I began to sleep at night and gradually began to come back to some sense of normalcy so that I could help take care of him and his brother.

My twelve-year-old needed me the most because he had known his mother and his uncles but still did not understand the magnitude of death. Thank God, he had always spent a great deal of time with us prior to his mother's death. Ryan never knew his mother. He was seventeen months old when she died and he had been in our care since he was born. I thank God that we gained permanent custody of our grandsons prior to their mother's death because it made it easier for us to maneuver and not worry about their dad complicating matters after her death. We advertised in the newspaper that we were seeking permanent custody but there was no response because they were in their own world; therefore probate court terminated their parental rights.

The children's deaths took some strange twists and turns. For instance, Valarie's small intestines twisted after she gave birth to Ryan via C-section. I have since learned that the small intestine always twists during a C-section but they usually go back into place. Also, the small intestines are usually attached to the stomach wall. In Valarie's case, her small intestines were not attached. Her small intestines swung freely and during the birthing process they twisted but did not untwist, thereby blocking blood flow through her organs. The blockage affected her small intestines, large intestines and part of her colon; all of which were surgically removed. After the surgery she was given a 50-50 chance of surviving. The blockage is called a volvulus. I heard the word "volvulus" and wondered, what in the world is that? It is not as though I understood medical terminology. Nevertheless, Valarie had to be fed through a feeding tube for the duration of her life. She lived in the hospital for seventeen months prior to her death.

WE NEED TO OPERATE ON VALARIE

THE TELEPHONE RANG ON MY SIDE OF THE BED AT 7:00 A.M. I PICKED IT UP AND SAID HELLO. A DESPERATE VOICE ON THE OTHER END ASKED FOR ME. I SAID, "YES, THIS IS SHE!" THE VOICE SAID, "MRS. JONES, YOU NEED TO COME TO THE HOSPITAL RIGHT AWAY. WE NEED TO OPERATE ON VALARIE. SHE NEEDS A HYSTERECTOMY RIGHT AWAY AND WE NEED YOUR SIGNATURE" (She had divorced her husband by this time and I was the next of kin)!

I asked, "What do you mean? I was just there last night and she was fine."

"Just come" the voice on the other end shouted! I awakened my husband to inform him that something was going on with Valarie at the hospital and they needed me to sign a permission form right away. I jumped into my clothes and sped to the hospital some fifteen miles away, praying and crying, "Lord, have mercy on my baby!"

I arrived at the hospital to find that she had been moved into intensive care. The plan was to stabilize her before she was operated on but by the time I arrived there was no time.

Valarie was in a room with very bright lights and tubes running from her body and a half dozen doctors and nurses all around her bed. When I walked in, a nurse said, "Thank God, you're here," and shoved a document into my hand to sign. The chief of staff looked at me and said, "We wanted to wait to stabilize her before operating but there is no time."

My mind was swirling and I wanted to scream at the doctors, "How did my daughter come to this hospital to give birth and end up in this condition? What have you done to her?" I needed answers but there were no answers. They would only say, "I am sorry but her condition changed!" But forty-eight hours ago she had given birth to a son by C-section. I saw her last night. What could have changed? We observed that her abdomen was extremely distended but we were told that it sometimes happened after a C-section. The rebel in me wanted answers. What happened to my daughter? But I said nothing, and the nurses rolled her down the hall and into the operating room while I stood there looking puzzled. The doctor looked back at me and promised to keep me updated. I slowly walked back to the waiting room, crying my heart out and that is where my pastor and his wife arrived and found me. He very sternly instructed me to go wash my face and comb my hair. He said, "She is going to need to see you holding it together when she comes out of surgery." I went into the bathroom to wash my face and comb my hair. My pastor's wife accompanied me into the bathroom. Just as we were coming out, one of her attending doctors came out of the operating room and said, "It was not her uterus, it was something else, but her doctor will be out to talk to you in a minute." By this time I was frantic and my pastor once again reminded me to be strong and to ask God for help. I really wanted to tell him to just "shut up!" The rebel in me wanted to ask him how he expected me to be strong when I did not know what was going on with my baby! Of course I did not say what I was feeling, I just sat there shaking and sniffling. Shortly thereafter, my husband arrived with Gerald and his cousin, Jason (Ryan was in the neo-natal unit in Yale New Haven Hospital some 45 miles away because he had become ill after birth (Where are you, God?). He was eventually diagnosed with Galactosemia. I asked his attending nurse, "What in the world is galactosemia?"

Here I go again, thrown into the world of foreign medical terms. In Ryan's case, his body could not and would not ever be able to break down milk or its derivatives (no milk, no cheese, no butter, no chocolate, etc.). He had become ill from the milk that was being fed to him following his birth and he had to be transported to Yale University Hospital and placed in the neonatal unit where he was tested to determine why he had become ill several days after his birth. I had to ask God if this was some kind of joke. How could Ryan and his mother be in critical care in hospitals 45 miles apart? God had to give me strength because I had to run between the two hospitals, while Basil cared for Gerald and our two businesses.

It seemed as though all hell had broken loose in my life.

My pastor was talking to Basil when the doctor came out with the bad news that it was a volvulus. He said, "We had to remove all of her small intestine, most of her large intestine, her colon and her bowels because they were gangrenous." OK, now I really needed answers. I needed to get to the truth of the matter. Did they mean that they had let my daughter lie in the hospital for 48 hours with every indication that her metabolism had changed and all they thought to do was bring in a psychiatrist. And now she had gangrene ravaging her internal organs.

A 50-50 CHANCE

I HEARD THE doctor say, "She has a fifty-fifty chance of surviving." I don't remember anything after that. But later I found myself sitting by her bedside. That was the day that I began descending into the abyss. That was the day that a part of my soul died. I could not tell night from day until my precious baby girl came out of an induced coma.

When she came out of the coma, she said, "Mommy," and I leaped from the chair where I had been keeping vigil, and I said, "I am right here, baby. I am right here." One tear cascaded down the side of her face. She didn't know what had happened to her. She was on a life support system with tubes running everywhere, and she looked at me whispering, "Mommy, where am I, where is my baby?"

I wiped her tears away and I stroked her brow and said, "Hush baby, just rest, sweetheart." I could not tell her that her baby had been moved to Yale New Haven Infant and Child Care Hospital. She would never know that her beloved baby had become very ill.

THE STORMS KEPT
ON COMING

AT THAT TIME Ryan had not been diagnosed with galactosemia. His condition was something we would learn about weeks down the road. As I stated, Galactosemia is a disease that a child is born with wherein their body is unable to break down milk or milk derivatives. Galactosemia can cause cataracts, liver failure and a host of other problems. After his birth, he was fed milk and it was making him very ill. He was rushed to a hospital 45 miles away and I began my trek from where we lived to two hospitals. Valarie in Stamford hospital and Ryan in Yale in New Haven. Somewhere in between I saw my husband and eldest grandson.

In the midst of Valarie's sickness, my husband had a heart attack and was hospitalized. He was in another wing of the same hospital as Valarie, and Ryan was still far away. God was carrying me because I could not have done it without Him. He kept me through all of the sicknesses that had penetrated my home, my heart, and my soul! I kept remembering the Psalms of David--the 23rd Psalm which is a beautiful and magnificent expression of my simple trust in God. When I uttered, "The Lord is my shepherd, I shall not want," I needed only to get to the verse which says, 'Thou restoreth my soul…" I knew that this was the epitome of God's grace when I journeyed into the abyss with a soul that was torn asunder. I knew that only God could restore my soul.

My husband recovered and the baby was brought home to a live-in sitter. God just showed up to take care of both of them. Still my soul needed restoring because my darling baby girl lingered in the hospital fighting off one infection after another and still had to be fed through a feeding tube into her stomach because she derived no nutritional value from the foods that she ate. She did not have intestines to process food. She did however still have tastes for some of her favorite foods from time to time. It was heartbreaking to know that when she had a taste for some of those favorite foods, none of it would help her nutritionally. But because she had gone through so much and had a life relegated to the hospital, we indulged her with the things that she desired.

After eight months of being in the hospital, Valarie insisted on going home to try to take care of her baby. We begged her doctor to let us take her home, and he did. He allowed her to go home for the weekend. However, she became very ill from a mishandling of her feeding tube. She picked up a very bad infection on the first day at home and almost died. Her doctor said emphatically that it would be a very long time before she would be able to go home again because we did not have the capability of taking care of her at home. From that point on everyone made a conscious effort to be more vigilant about spending time with her at the hospital. Her brothers, other family members, her friends, church members and so many others made a pact to make sure someone was there every day. And, we made a point of taking the children to visit her more often. The baby did not know her so we had a hard time getting him to visit with her. He was spoiled rotten by his grandfather but she took pride in saying, "I can't wait to get home so I can un-spoil you."

She did not know it, but our plan was to build an extension on our home if she recovered, so she would have her own apartment. We had no intention of letting the children out of our sight. We also knew that she could not care for the children alone. In fact, she could not care for them at all because her feeding tube would be her constant companion. At that time they were not doing intestinal transplants. Today intestinal transplants are possible. In fact, there are centers all over the world that do intestinal transplants. It has become more commonplace as more and more research has gone into repairing complete blockages and obstructions of the intestines and the bowels. At the time, there was no hope for Valarie's condition. Transplantation of the intestines was still being researched.

HELP MY UNBELIEF

OVER THE SEVENTEEN-MONTH period that Valarie lived in the hospital, she developed a number of illnesses that kept her bouncing back and forth from a regular hospital room to intensive care. She developed pneumonia, a gall bladder infection, and an infection of the hip that ate into her hip bone. Each one of these illnesses set her back a month or more. When the infection in her hip set in, it was ignored until she could no longer walk. The nurses complained about her unwillingness to walk; she complained that it hurt too much. But this interaction taught me something. I learned that no one can tell you about someone else's pain. Whenever someone tells me that another person could not possibly be in that much pain, the rebel in me rises to the surface and I cut them off at the pass.

My daughter made a believer out of me because from the time they operated on her hip she never walked again. I blame the hospital for having to operate on her. It was sheer negligence because her complaints were ignored. Instead of ruling out problems that would hinder her ability to walk, the nurses complained that she would not get out of the bed. When I asked Valarie why she would not get up and walk around, she said, "Mommy, it just hurts too much!"

I told the nurses what she said and they looked at me as if to say, "There is no reason why she should be in pain."

Time would prove that their assumptions were wrong, and she would end up having surgery on her hip because of an inflammation in the hip bone. She began to go downhill after the surgery because the infection had spread throughout her body. It had gotten so bad on the day she was rushed back into intensive care, a nurse who had gone to school with Valarie found my number and called to tell me that I needed to make the hospital tell me what was going on with her. On that same day, one of the doctors called to say that they were rushing her into intensive care. I rushed to the hospital to find her hooked up to life support and in an induced coma, once again. I purposed in my mind that I would watch over her all day every day for as long as she lived. No one would have to call me to say that her condition had changed because I would be there with her no matter what.

My "no matter what" attitude took a toll on my private life. My husband complained to others that I was never home, that I was neglecting the business that I was responsible for, that I did not spend time with him or the boys. But, I did not concerned about the business nor him, even though he was right. I was not going to leave her. This rebel had a cause.

DANCING WITH MY BABY

HER CONDITION HAD worsened and she remained in intensive care on life support. I knew that the end was near so I instructed the babysitter and family members to make sure that my eldest grandson's Christmas was as normal as possible. I did not want his life disrupted if his mother passed away during the holidays. Ryan was only sixteen months old and did not know anything about Christmas. But I came home at night from the hospital and danced with him in my arms to the sounds of "Kenny G." Kenny G's music helped me make it through the long days and nights. Holding Valarie's baby and dancing with him close gave me comfort. Holding him close helped me make it through the night, not knowing what to expect in the morning. I held him because I knew that I would never hold his mother again. In him, I could smell her. In him, I could imagine what her body felt like as he lay in her womb. In him, I could experience her soul. He was the last to be connected to her. I needed his closeness to help me make it to the end. I danced with Ryan every night until the end. I danced with him and I prayed that God would be merciful and take her to another place with Him where there would be no more pain and no more suffering. I danced with him with a heavy heart as I sought God on behalf of my daughter who had been lingering and suffering day and night for seventeen months with no relief. My cry was, "Lord, have mercy on my child! Lord, have mercy on me!" It was not long after I began my dance routine with the baby when one of her doctors asked me if I wanted her revived if her heart stopped. The rebel in me rose up and I said, "No, leave her alone; if her heart stops, let her go. She has had enough!"

She had already told me prior to the infection that she was tired. She looked at me one day prior to going into intensive care for the third or fourth time and said, "Mommy, I am just tired."

I looked at her, trying to hold back tears, and I said, "Baby, if you are tired, just go to sleep. If you are concerned about the children, don't worry, we will take good care of them."

These were my babies. She did not have to worry. I would never let anything happen to her darling sons. She had been suffering long enough. I did not want to prolong her suffering even though it was breaking my heart to tell her that it was OK to leave her precious children and me. That was the last conversation that I had with her even though she lived three or four weeks after that conversation. I say she lived but it was not really living; she existed on life support for an additional three or four weeks. A machine kept her alive while we waited for her heart to stop.

I had already been prepped about what it meant to have a "quality life." This young nurse pulled me to the side one day to inform me that the doctor would eventually ask me what I wanted to do when her heart stopped. She said, "They are going to ask you about reviving her. I cannot tell you what to do but please think about what her quality of life would be like if she is brought back. She is going to be on a feeding tube for the rest of her life and she will not be able to care for her children." The nurse turned around to look at me as she said, "Mrs. Jones, I really do not think that your daughter would want to live like that."

The rebel in me wanted to ask her, 'How in the world would you know what my daughter would want?' I wanted to ask her what gave her the right to even talk to me about my daughter. I wanted to lash out at her and tell her, "You don't know my daughter like that."

Instead I listened without commenting. She said, "Ask the doctor how long she will live and what condition will she be in if she is revived?" I listened to the nurse without commenting because I knew that Valarie had endured so many setbacks and she had already told me that she was tired. Not only that, sepsis had set in; she had an infection that had eaten away her hip bone and may have sent her body into septic shock. When the doctor approached me about reviving her, I said, "No thank you, sir. She has had enough."

Why would I resuscitate her when the prognosis was so negative? I asked the doctor how long she would survive if she was resuscitated and he said, "A couple of days or maybe even a week and then we would have to do it again." She was young enough to survive resuscitation if she had not had pneumonia and other health issues, but her body was in no condition to sustain further beatings. I looked at her and said, "Just leave her alone! She is tired and has told me that she just can't take it anymore!" My baby girl had suffered beyond anyone's imagination. Her life had been relegated to hospital beds, feeding tubes, and pain. She was ready to go and I had prepared myself to let her go.

PERVERSION IN
THE HOSPITAL

VALARIE'S PROGNOSIS WAS not good when she went into intensive care even though her body did not look beaten up. The edema that would take over her body and cause disfiguration had not set in. She looked perfectly normal and that is the reason why I was about to beat a male nurse down. I walked into her room one day and found her beautiful thighs and legs uncovered up to her pelvic area while he bounced around her room doing whatever. I looked at him and asked just one simple question, "Why is she uncovered like that?"

That pervert looked at me with fear in his eyes and said, "I just finished giving her a bath." Really! "Well, you are not bathing her now! Cover her up and you can get out of here. I will be with her for the rest of the day!"

I guess no one told him that I was there each and every day. Had he known, I suspect that he would have been more discreet with his perversion. I reported the pervert and told the head nurse that I did not want him back in her room and he was never to touch her again. l looked the head nurse dead in her face, and said, "She might be on life support, but I am not; my daughter will leave here with her dignity intact." She made some lame excuse but the pervert never came back into her room again.

I was at the hospital every day. And one day a member of our church who worked at the hospital stopped by to see how Valarie was doing. She asked me if I came and just sat every day. I responded, "Yes, I do. She knows that I am here!" For me that was all that really mattered. She knew that I was sitting by her bedside. Nothing else mattered; not even my upset husband who complained about me spending all of my time at the hospital. Rebels have to do what rebels have to do. We do not care what anybody says. I tried not to be offensive, but for goodness sake leave me alone! For me, Valarie had already crossed over. I saw her dying and I had no intention of letting her die alone. I planned on being there with her when she drew her last breath. I sat with her day in and day out. When her heart finally stopped, I was right there watching as it all came to an end. I was sitting on my husband's lap as we watched her heart rate slowly drop. By this time, he also knew that the end was near and he no longer complained to his friends about the time that I spent at the hospital. He joined me as often as he could. And we were there together when she "flatlined."

A REBEL'S CRY

I SAW IT happening, but when her heart finally stopped, my piercing cry could be heard throughout ICU. I CRIED, "LORD, HAVE MERCY ON ME" and then blacked out! When I came to, my husband and a nurse were standing over me. He was calling me by my nickname; "BJ, BJ, it is going to be all right, honey!" No, it would never be alright again. I walked around like a zombie; unable to eat, sleep, or care for the boys. Thank God for live-in help. Thank God for my husband. I was a basket case! Our live-in help was the best thing that ever happened to my family. She cooked, cleaned, and delicately took care of the boys. She witnessed Ryan taking his first steps. I was in and out of the house so I missed important things like first steps; but she was always happy to show off his developmental stages. The only thing that I could do was pick Ryan up, dance around the room to Kenny G, give him a hug and a kiss, and tell him how much I loved him. Gerald was almost nine years old when his mother died, so he moved quietly around either doing homework or playing with his toys until his cousin and the twins came to live with us. Somehow his cousin mysteriously showed up, not that I minded because he was good company for Gerald. They were close in age. I just cannot remember a conversation about the prospect of us taking care of him. I guess the assumption was that one more did not matter because we had a helper. But then three became five and there was no mystery to how that happened.

We became parents to two foster children as part of our family about a year or so after Valarie's death. They were ten years old. The boy had cerebral palsy and the little girl was mentally disturbed. She had been sold into prostitution at the age of eight and she suffered from mental illness as a result of what she had experienced at the hands of her drug-addicted mother. It was a strange situation, because at first, her twin brother had to be taken to visit his mother in prison at least once a month but the girl was not allowed to have contact with her. But, as time progressed, the girl began to cry and scream each time her brother went off for a day to visit their mother. Finally, her psychiatrist gave permission for her to go on supervised visits to see her mother along with her brother.

In the beginning of her visits, I had to accompany the social worker with the children on visits to see their mother because the girl did not want to go without me. In retrospect, I guess she was afraid that I might not want her to come back to our home if she showed too much love for her mother. The girl child was anxious to reassure me that I was really her mother because the woman in prison had let men do awful things to her. She told me how her mother prepared her for men by soaking her in the bath tub, putting perfume and lipstick on her. It tore my heart out of my chest to hear what had happened to this beautiful ten-year-old child. I could only say, "You are safe now." Oddly enough, each time that I went with the children to visit their mother, she thanked me for taking care of her children and for keeping them together. She always added "for keeping them together" because they were about to be separated when we stepped up, offering our hearts, our love, and the safety of a home devoid of treachery and wrongdoing. We offered the children a place called home. I suppose someone told the mother what her children were facing before we became involved.

When we heard the plight of the children, I begged my husband to let us take them. At first he was reluctant to even talk about it but I cried all afternoon and he finally said it was ok for me to check and find out what the requirements were. We had two extra bedrooms so space was not a problem. When he said check out the requirements, I was elated! I called Family and Children services the very next day and was told what we needed to do to qualify to become foster parents. It was a process that I eagerly agreed to because I wanted to make a home for these two lovely children. I alone went to the classes, my husband did not. Although both of us were supposed to attend classes together, that is where he drew the line. But we had a lovely supportive social worker who was gracious enough to come to our home to interview him. When she came to our home, she said quietly, "I need some place to stay." We were approved immediately and the day the children were brought to our home by the social worker was one of the happiest days I had experienced in a very long time. We ended up caring for four boys and one girl. It was not easy caring for so many children, but most of the children could care for themselves when it came to things like taking a bath, and even doing their homework, and, of course we still had a live-in sitter.

I loved shopping for the little girl. I loved taking her to church so that I could show her off. She was a blessing even though she was mentally messed up because of the ordeal that she had been through. In many ways she was dangerous because she had promiscuous tendencies and on occasion she would approach adult men and tell them that they could do whatever they wanted to do to her. She went as far as telling them that she would not tell anybody. When I heard this, I knew that I had to take her with me if the babysitter was off for the day and our grown sons or their friends were around.

If you approached her about her tendencies she denied it and would scream to the top of her lungs. Interestingly enough, she was beloved by everyone in the neighborhood. She was adorable and outgoing. She met people on our street that we had never met. But again, she had to be watched. She was not allowed to ride her bike out of sight without her brothers accompanying her. We were afraid of what might happen to her. Her twin brother, on the other hand, was very calm. He dared not do anything that might cause him to be removed from the comfort of his home, and he hated it when his sister got into trouble. The only thing that he desired was his food, the privacy of his room, television, visits with his mother, and an occasional visit with his father. He did spend some time with the other boys though he could not keep up when they played outside. But he loved it when they were relegated to playing or watching TV in the basement because of the weather. He was not completely incapacitated by the cerebral palsy; he simply walked with a bad limp and only had use of one arm.

Everything was going along fine until we decided to relocate to Georgia. I needed to get away from the pain that still gripped my heart after Valarie's death. When the doctors informed my husband that he would not survive the brutal winters of the North with the condition of his heart, both of us were happy and ready to relocate. He wanted to go back home to Jamaica but I said no way. I was not going to raise my grandchildren in Jamaica so I suggested Atlanta and he agreed. We both acknowledged that our Home Heating Oil business sometimes kept him outside all night during the winter months and he could not continue with the business. The major problem was the work that we sometimes had to do with government contracts would always be difficult. The contracts included providing heating oil to government buildings but also required maintenance of the heating units. If a unit broke down during the night we were required to have it up and running before office hours the next day. Sometimes it took all night to repair or replace a heating unit and he would be up all night in the cold making sure that the work was done so that government employees would not be inconvenienced. It had gotten to be difficult for him and we could not find dependable help to oversee that end of the business. We tried leasing it out before we made the final decision to close it down.

Another reason for closing the business down had to do with the federal government and its ruling that all in-ground oil tanks had to be either taken up or filled with some substance that I cannot recall, and no matter which way we went, it was going to cost a fortune. We decided to let it go because the person leasing the business wanted to be able to utilize the in-ground tanks but they could not. We opted to do nothing even though we owned the building to which the tanks were attached. Our first concern was my husband's health and of course my sanity, and not the business. When we migrated to Georgia we left owning a business that we could do nothing with and three children whose hearts were broken.

The twins were wards of the State until they turned eighteen years old. However, they could not move with us because neither of their parents had been denied parental rights. Somewhere along the way, child welfare had decided that the boy still needed his mom in his life. So, they could only live with us in Connecticut. I hated losing them but I needed space between me and the heartbreak of knowing and being reminded by others of the grave (that would become three in the future and were within close proximity to me no matter where I went). If I was ever going to come back from the abyss I had to separate myself from the grave, and the questions and the looks that said, "I feel sorry for you!"

IF I COULD DANCE WITH
MY BABY AGAIN

NO ONE COULD have prepared me for the loss of another child. That was too far-fetched to believe. First my daughter, and now my youngest son; no way! William was an unusual young man. He was handsome, debonair, socially astute and an avid reader. He dropped out of college (rather, got suspended because he spent all of his time playing cards during his first and second semesters of college). Afterward, he still walked around in a suit jacket, khakis, a shirt and tie, and a newspaper under his arm. That suit jacket and tie with a newspaper opened a lot of doors for him. He was hired for some of the best and highest paying jobs available. He wasn't just carrying the newspaper; he actually read the newspaper. He read it from front to back every day and could talk about any newsworthy subject matter. He was a "rebel without a cause" until his sister died. She had spoiled him rotten. He was her baby!

Her death shook him to the core of his soul. He even blamed the baby for her death, not knowing that she planned it because she had always wanted another child. Billy loved her as much as she loved him. No matter what he did, she was always there for him. I was happy to see that his routine did not change after his sister's death. He still walked around dressed up with his newspaper under his arm. Sometime during the day, he would read the newspaper from front to cover.

We learned that he loved reading the newspapers while he was in high school. One of his teachers discovered his love for reading newspapers because he caught him reading it every chance that he got. If he was allowed to read the newspaper, he would do anything that his teacher asked him to do. He graduated from high school with honors--not as the valedictorian or salutatorian—but as the young person who had made the greatest strides. He gave a speech in which he thanked everybody for seeing the best in him. I had never been more proud of him than at that moment.

Billy went off to college at my insistence but, as I said, he did not do well because he spent all of his time playing cards instead of studying. When he returned home, he began dating a lovely young girl who was as sweet as she could be, and they became the parents of two lovely children, a boy and a girl. I thought that everything was going well between the two of them, but then it seemed as though their relationship just fell apart. I blamed him totally for the breakup because I am not sure that he ever grew up. He was moving her and the children every six months from one place to another. They even spent some time living at home. But I had given him a time limit to get his life in order and when it was up, he had to have saved enough money to take care of his family. Of course that never happened and shortly thereafter, we migrated to Atlanta and he ended up with another girl who he eventually married and it was sometime after this marriage that his life ended. I never asked him or his former love what happened even though my grandchildren's lives hung in the balance. But his former love has taken good care of them with the help of her parents. His son looks and acts just like him and the daughter looks exactly like her mother (except for her feet. She has flat feet like her father and I). I have a total of 4 grandchildren and 3 great grandchildren and I love all of them from the depths of my soul. They have given me my life back. They have given me the zeal to come back from the abyss.

Billy did some crazy things in his life. Sometimes, even now, I walk by his picture and smile, saying to his picture, "You were one crazy kid." I recall how he wrestled with his son and his nephews before we migrated to Georgia. I would tell him to stop because he seemed so rough, but they would squeal with delight encouraging him to do whatever he was doing again. I would say stop, and they would say, "Do it again, Uncle Billy" or "Do it again, Daddy." They loved rough-housing with him, so I finally gave up.

I have asked "Why God?" because I really needed Jesus to walk with me through this dark and dreary place. Billy's death sent me into an unbelievable tailspin that caused me to descend back into a place from which I thought that I had escaped.

The last time I saw my baby boy alive, I danced with him at his wedding. He had just married a young woman that he met in a town nearby. They dated for about a year before he asked her to marry him. They were married in September and he disappeared in October. His new bride did not report him missing, nor did she report her car missing. She said, "I thought he had decided to move to Georgia with you."

Now why would your new husband move to Georgia with his mother? And why didn't you try to find him? Lord, I need you to hold my hand. I am trying to figure this all out and it smells like the new wife is hiding something. "I believe,' Lord help my unbelief." I danced with my baby at his wedding—a joyous occasion, and now I am descending back into the dark pits of hell because he is nowhere to be found. I had to ask God once again, to "have mercy on me." It seemed as though everything in my life was spiraling out of control. Whispering a prayer of faith, I flew to New York on my way to Connecticut in search of my baby boy. I said over and over again, "Lord, I trust you.' Lord I love you, 'Lord I trust you, 'Lord I love you, 'Lord, please let my baby be ok." I didn't know what else to say or do. I felt that if I did not keep talking to God, I was going to lose it before I arrived in New York. I made it to New York and my now deceased oldest son and Billy's best friend picked me up at the airport with the bad news. William had not been seen since the night he went to pick his wife up from work and she had to work overtime. According to her, "William came to pick me up but I had to work another hour. I told him to come back in an hour but he never came back."

"Lord, have mercy on me?" At this point, William had been missing for over a month. We went to the police department but there was no record of a missing person report or a missing car report ever being filed. This I thought was very strange. We didn't know anything about this young woman. We didn't know how they met, or anything. We were at a complete loss because our hands were tied. We turned over every rock in the two weeks that I was there but nothing came up that would help us. I prayed to God that he had decided to just take off. But deep down in my heart, I knew that something bad had happened to my baby and I did not know if I could take it when it was revealed to me. After two weeks, I returned to Georgia not knowing any more about the whereabouts of my baby than I had when I left.

I went back to Georgia carrying the weight of a missing son and the knowledge that I had buried a daughter in Connecticut. I carried the weight of running away from the pain of my daughter's death and now a greater weight was on my shoulders that said I should not have moved so far away from him. I felt as though I had deserted him. I blamed myself for not being there. I blamed myself for his marrying someone that we did not know. Maybe I could have protected him if I had not moved so far away. I began to search for him in crowds on television, on the streets, at a basketball game, or wherever crowds gathered. I saw him everywhere, but I did not see him anywhere. Everybody looked like him but nobody was him. Every time the telephone rang, I prayed that I would hear his voice on the other end. Lord, if I could just hear his voice, if I could see his face, if I could just laugh at his antics, if I could dance with my baby again!

I was on an emotional roller coaster when the call came six months after I returned to Georgia. His body had been found by a river bank by a woman walking her dog. His body was badly decomposed from being out in the elements all winter long.

I had been praying for closure but not like this. I had been praying day and night that God would reveal to me his whereabouts. I lost interest in everything and everybody. I could not focus. This was a blank dark period for me. I descended head first into the beyond. The only thing that I can recall about those six months was my obsession with finding my baby boy. God, I yearned to dance with my baby again; but it was not to be. Winter came and went. It was Springtime when he was found. It was after the snow-covered grounds of Connecticut had thawed. Nature lovers could walk through the woods again. It was on a walk through the woods toward the river that my baby boy's body was found. He was slumped over a table with his coat covering his head. My dearly beloved baby boy was dead; cause unknown. My God, my God, why have you forsaken me? This was more than I could take. I was inconsolable; and I lost all sense of time and space. I guess the wife who did not care enough about him to report him missing, made the funeral arrangements. The only thing that I can recall is sitting in a strange church. The funeral was not held in my former church because she wanted it held in her church. I do recall sitting in the hotel talking to my former pastor and I said to him, "This is not about my children; this is about me. The devil is after my soul but he cannot have it."

His response was odd for a pastor. He simply said, "I don't know now!" He may not have known but I knew without a doubt that the devil had come to steal, kill and destroy. I also knew that by plucking my children off one by one, the devil wanted me to "curse God and die." But I had a faith like Job and I said to myself, "I will not go down like this!" I don't remember much else but I remember the conversation and I remember that I had to be a strong tower of faith. Everything else is pretty blank. I cannot recall going to Connecticut for the funeral nor do I recall going back home to Georgia. Because of my mental state, I was medicated then and in the months to come. I was a zombie! I moved around like a lifeless doll. The only time that I came to life was when my oldest son called. He could always make me smile because he had an infectious laugh.

SOME KIND OF A JOKE

CHARLES HAD A deep belly laugh and he could always make me laugh. He knew how deep the pain was for me to lose his brother and his sister. We did not talk about Valarie or Billy's deaths very often. We kind of skirted around Billy's death in particular because ultimately we would end with the conclusion that Billy's wife had him murdered. We could not say why but the rebel in me believes that she had him murdered because the evidence seemed to point in her direction. I repeat, she did not try to find him and she never called either one of us. And had it not been for his best friend inquiring about him and bringing it to his brother's attention and later to my attention, we would have gone on thinking that he was living in wedded bliss and did not have time for us.

All of this thinking about his death has me weighted down until this day. And I am like a lot of African American women, I am burdened down by mental illness but my use of mental health services is zero.

I am still angry at Charles for leaving me. Every time I spoke to him, I said, "Son, please take care of yourself. You know you are all that I have left."

I wonder sometimes whether I worried him to death with the constant begging and pleading. I know that it sounds crazy but I thought that if I reminded him that he was all that I had, he would be careful. Of course, God's plan is not our plan. On the night of his death, I could not sleep. I was sitting on the side of the bed with the TV still playing and Basil turned over and said, "BJ, please turn the TV off and come to bed."

I said, "OK honey, I am!"

I turned the TV off and climbed into bed but I began to toss and turn. Somewhere near 3:00 am the phone rang and a voice on the other end, said, "Betty, put Basil on the phone." I said to the person at the other end, "He's asleep."

They very roughly said, "Betty, I said put Basil on the phone."

I said "OK" because I knew deep down in my soul something had happened to Charles. I shook him and said, "Someone wants to speak to you," and I handed him the phone. I heard him say calmly, "OK, we will leave in the morning."

I asked him what was going on but he did not have the heart to tell me that my last child was dead. He said, "Charles is in the hospital in Massachusetts and we have to go to him." I was panic-stricken and screamed, "What happened to him?"

He said, "I don't know, BJ. We just have to go. Please lay back down and try to sleep so we can make arrangements to go to him tomorrow." When the call came, Charles was already dead. He died at the hands of the police from strangulation. Basil knew but he could not speak the words that would shatter my world to pieces.

Two weeks prior to that call, I had danced with my eldest son one last time. We attended a family wedding and he was one of the groomsmen. He was dressed in a peach tuxedo and boy was he looking good. He asked me if I was having fun as we danced the evening away. It had only been thirteen and one half months since we found his brother's body and I knew that he was asking me if I was having fun, because it had not been that long since I danced with his brother at his wedding. I tried to have fun but my heart was not in it. We talked about his decision not to come to Georgia on his vacation this year because we were spending the week in Connecticut. Even though it made sense, I was terribly disappointed that he would not be coming to Georgia. He came to visit every year and we loved it. The boys looked forward to his visit.

Charles was the one child that I could depend on. If I was ill he would come and sit by my bedside. Sometimes he slept, but he was there. He had always been the caring child. I could always count on him, though we did have our issues.

For instance, I came home from work unexpectedly and found that he and a bunch of his buddies had skipped school and were holed up in his room smoking marijuana and I threatened to kill all of them. He also did things to drive his sister crazy when she tried to keep the house clean to take the burden off of me.

She would clean the house and he would come along and mess it up and it erupted into an argument that wasn't very pretty. And I cannot count the number of times that I had to go to school for meetings because he just would not do his school-work. How he made it out of high school I do not know. In fact, I do not know how he kept a relationship with a woman either (or did he?). One of his girlfriends said that he was a practicing Muslim and wanted her to walk behind him. Another said he was too possessive; so I really do not know. I know that he drove his sister crazy when they were growing up. That was Charles, my eldest son.

Valarie was a neat freak and Charles was a slob--that is until he rented his own apartment. I could not believe my eyes when I walked into his apartment. The place was so clean I could not believe that it belonged to him. Not a thing out of place. Not even a dirty glass in the sink. He even had the nerve to walk behind me whenever I visited him, picking up things. I had to ask myself on several occasions if this was the same boy who left empty pizza boxes under his bed? Duh! Well, yeah! After all, he entertained females in his apartment. And check this out--no one could just walk up to his apartment unannounced. He lived in one of those fancy secured apartment buildings at this sought-after address.

My son had a nice apartment, a nice car, and a great job. My son had arrived! He was working at one of those Fortune 500 compa-nies, traveled where he wanted to and had a great life. He loved the life he lived and lived the life he loved. It was there on one of his trips that he met his untimely death struggling with the police after some craziness at a basketball court. Autopsy revealed an old heart (he was 29 years old) of a 65-year-old man, and strangulation. He was not married so the police got away with murder. By this time, I was too mentally exhausted to fight! I just wanted the Last Dance. Three children dead in five years! Lord, help!

YOU HAVE GOT TO
BE KIDDING

GOD HAS A funny way of doing things. I was walking around in a zombie-like state wondering what I did to cause God to be so angry at me that he would take all three of my children. And here comes God waking me up every morning at 3:30am like an alarm clock with instructions to tell the world that He loved them. At first I said, "God, you have got to be kidding! You want me to tell people that you love them when I don't even feel loved."

What I should have said was, "God, you got jokes!" But I simply said, "I have no platform to tell anybody anything." That did not stop God from waking me up every morning at the same time with the same instructions. It was not until I went to my pastor to tell him that I believed God was calling me into the ministry that God stopped waking me up at 3:30 am. My pastor made a joke about my "Call" so I cut the conversation off as I said to myself, this is going nowhere so I will just forget it.

I did what I was supposed to do and I will leave the rest up to God. But God was not kidding, nor did God have jokes. Almost four months to the date of my son's death, here comes death again! It happened when I took my husband to his cardiologist for an examination and he was rushed from the doctor's office to the hospital for open heart surgery. This is where God showed me off to my pastor. My husband was in surgery for 7 ½ hours (a 3 ½ hour surgery) and he died three times. Everything stopped. No pulse, no heartbeat, no brain signals, nothing! I did not know what was going on so every hour after the 3 ½ hours I was told that it would take, I sent my pastor to the nurse's station in an attempt to find out what was happening. The answer was always the same, "They are still in surgery." My pastor was getting on my last nerve with, "No news is good news!" I was in no mood for clichés. I wanted to know what was going on with my husband. I had just buried the last of my three children. My nerves were on edge. The chaplain came to get me 7 and 1/2 hours later. He came up to me and said, "Mrs. Jones, the doctor would like to talk to you."

I looked up at him but turned to my pastor and said, "I told you he was dead."

The chaplain very gently said, "The doctor just needs to talk to you." He could not say more. I was taken into a private waiting room to hear the bad news that they were not sure whether he would make it through the night. They had lost him on the operating table three times but they kept working on him looking for answers. Everything worked when they took the heart out of his chest but as soon as they placed it back into the heart cavity, everything in his body shut down. The doctor kept working on him and they found that he was allergic to a blood thinner after three tries (I was told that they usually only try twice, then they give up). So here we were with the bad news that he may not make it. The doctor looked at me, not my pastor, and said, "If you have a relationship with God, I suggest you start praying." He said, "He will be coming by soon; you may see him and touch him but he is out of it. Just pray. When the doctor walked out I asked my pastor to call the prayer warrior from church but he could not find her. After several failed attempts, I began to pray. I did not ask my pastor to pray but I myself began to call on the name of Jesus on behalf of my husband. When I stopped praying, my pastor looked at me, and said, "If I did not know that you were 'called' before, I know it now." He said, "When Basil is better we will place you under watch care and begin your training toward pastoral ministry."

Basil survived the open heart surgery and lived another seven years. When he died he did not die from heart-related problems, but from pancreatic cancer. He continued to guide the lives of our grandsons as I continued on my journey in the academic world.

When he died, I was studying for a Doctor of Ministry degree. I earned the Masters of Divinity while he was alive. He was able to celebrate that accomplishment with me, and rightfully so because, through the movement of the Holy Spirit, he initiated the process in the first place.

I recall receiving an invitation to a ministry conference at the Interdenominational Theological Center and I wondered out loud where they got my contact information from. I railed against attending the three-day conference. I said to Basil, "I am not going to school with a bunch of "young things" right out of college. He said, "BJ, just call the school and get the details and then you can ask about the age of attendees." I was in for a surprise. The average age was the mid-forties but there were some attendees who were over seventy years old. "Well, shut the door!" I was not getting out of this thing. Basil said, "Ok, BJ, what is your excuse now? Why don't you go for one day; if you do not like it, just don't go back?"

I said, "Ok." So I went, and before the day was over, I was calling home shouting, "I am going to seminary!"

My sweet husband simply said, "That was quick." Thus began my seminary journey toward becoming a learned minister. I completed the MDIV with honors and was accepted into the Doctor of Ministry program the same year. I completed the DMIN program 2 ½ years later and was immediately hired as an adjunct professor in Ministry and Context at the ITC. I held that position for twelve years. During this same period I moved my membership from the Baptist denomination to United Methodist and within 1 ½ years, I was hired in a Methodist church as an associate pastor to jump start an emerging church. I remained in that position for fourteen months before being appointed senior pastor in the church that I now serve. While teaching at the seminary I was also hired as the director of Faith Journey, a mentoring program for 1st year seminarians and post graduate seminarians. God's plan for my ministerial life was unfolding in many places and quite rapidly.

PART II

COPING WITH SUFFERING

REBELS CAN BE so foolish! Did I really think that becoming a foster parent would help me get through some of the anguish of losing a daughter? The warning came that no one should try to replace a loved one with a foster child. It does not work! I wanted a little girl even though I was warned not to take one if I was attempting to fill a void caused by a personal loss. Although it was not the ultimate goal, it did help to have a little girl around again. I loved shopping for her, but a little piece of me had died with my daughter. Valarie's death really messed with my mind. I was messed up and everybody suffered. I did not deal with her death very well. And I did not seek the help that I so desperately needed. Sometimes I was so irrational it was beyond belief. For instance, I jumped up one day and decided that I needed to go to Hawaii. My husband asked me to wait a few weeks for him. I said, "I can't wait for a few weeks, I am going next week (we owned a travel agency)." He begged me to wait for a few weeks so we could go together; but I was not hearing it. I had to get away from it all right now. My dearly beloved daughter was gone and I had to get away from everything that was familiar to me. Rebels can be a little overzealous. I arrived in Honolulu, and I went straight to my hotel. As God would have it, my beautiful room overlooked the ocean. At night I left my balcony doors open and my soul was soothed by the waves splashing against the shore. There were evenings when my nephew, who resided in Honolulu, came by the hotel to have dinner with me. I had a marvelous time laughing at his jokes as we talked about old times especially our dinner table antics when we were younger; and how we used to grab for the last biscuit. It was so refreshing to have something to laugh about.

The entire trip was relaxing. During the day I wandered the island, going from shop to shop and stopping at quaint cafes for lunch. It was the best thing I could have done for myself. God arrested me in Honolulu and sent me back home to my family in a better state of mind.

Like most African American women, who are suffering from mental distress, I was closed to the idea of professional help. Most of the time, we are contradictions to the status quo. Some African Americans seek religious help from their pastor, but I did not. I suffered in silence. And although I suffered in silence, I came back from Hawaii better able to cope with my daughter's death. From the time my daughter went into surgery and subsequently died, I was an emotional wreck and felt that a soft wind could knock me over. During this time of mental anguish, anything could knock me over. The only help that I sought was that of my pastor on the day of her surgery; and the only thing that I asked him to do was to pray for me.

I realized that I needed someone to talk to when I began to feel a hatred inside of me that was not good. I hated my daughter's friends who were still alive. I could not understand why God took my child and left them here to torment me. My rationale was that she was a nice girl and did not deserve to die and perhaps God had made a mistake in taking her instead of them. With all of this venom inside of me, I still did not seek professional help; instead I sought healing through God. I cried and I prayed. I could not seek professional help even if I knew someone because individuals in the community would have said that I could not cope, that I'd had a nervous breakdown. I was determined not to let anyone think that I could not cope. After all I was a Black woman who was also a civil rights leader. Civil rights leaders had to be strong; Black women had to be strong. I had to handle myself correctly. I waved the banner, I challenged the systems, and I sat with CEOs and senators over lunch discussing matters affecting the community. These giant corporate leaders and the U.S. senator were guest speakers at NAACP dinners that I hosted. They filled the banquet halls with purchased tables, they directed a percentage of certain business components to my small businesses, and I was invited to participate in Small Business Initiatives (SBA). How could they know that while all of this was going on, inside I was an emotional wreck? I was an accident waiting to happen, but I still had to handle myself correctly. I had a reputation to maintain.

I did handle myself in the best way that I knew how. I walked the floor at night and I lay on the couch with a pillow over my head when I was away from the crowds. Everyone with whom I came in contact commented on my strength. They called me a modern day "Job!" I was no Job! I was dying inside but no one could see it. I was mentally depressed but I was in denial. And, mentally depressed or not, something had to change because I had three little boys and a set of twins to care for. I prayed and reminded God that he had given me these precious lives and I needed to be able to sleep at night so that I could care for them during the day. It was not fair to my husband or the live-in help. God heard my cry and I began to sleep at night but I was still an emotional wreck. Everything made me cry and I needed help to get through each day, but I did not seek it. Stigma that was so pervasive in the African American community was now my daily friend. Stigma had my address and I was letting it take me down.

I began forgetting appointments for my grandsons and the other children as well as for myself.

Somewhere along the way, I was reminded of a beautiful young woman who developed a mental illness because of a failed relationship. The separation devastated her to the point that she was unable to function. Separation of any kind can destroy you if you do not get a handle on it. This young lady was one of the most articulate and beautiful women I had ever known. Prior to her deterioration, she spoke at board of education meetings on behalf of the NAACP articulating the need to stop closing inner city schools. She went before the Fair Housing Commission to talk about the need for affordable housing in her community. But a failed relationship took her down. She could no longer hold a job because she could not remember what she was supposed to be doing and she ended up as a welfare recipient because of mental illness. I witnessed her deterioration and I saw first-hand what mental illness brought on by the loss of a loved one can do to a person. Her family did not seek professional help for her because of stigma. I was now faced with this same type of stigma, so I used religion but I would have been better served if I had sought professional help. I would have been better able to handle the next devastating blows that would take center stage in my life. I would have been better equipped to cope with suffering.

Many African American descend into the abyss; and some do not find their way back. It is the stigma associated with mental health that has kept me and countless other African American women from seeking help for their mental illness. Stigma has been identified as the most significant barrier to seeking mental health services among African Americans but very little attention has been given to examining stigma, the beliefs about mental illness that may be associated with stigma, and how these beliefs may affect our approach to coping.

Although I should have, I did not seek mental health services. It had nothing to do with the usual barriers, such as inaccessible location, transracial and ethnic minority clinicians, transportation problems, lack of health insurance, and poverty, nor availability of services (limited access to culturally competent clinicians and case management) and cultural matching few opportunities to work with racial and ethnic minority clinicians. I did not seek mental health services because of stigma. I did not want to be labeled as a "crazy" woman who lost her mind because her entire family was gone. I was fully aware that I was mentally depressed because I cried at the mention of my children's names; but I failed to address my illness. I was traumatized by my children's deaths. I am still traumatized and I still get emotional over the loss of my children, some twenty-three years later. Nobody has seen my tears because I do not allow anyone to ask me about their deaths. If I mention that they are deceased and someone asks for details, I simply say, "I don't care to talk about it."

Belief about mental illness, including stigma related to mental illness, are prevalent in society whether or not an individual has direct experience with mental illness or not. Thus, beliefs have the potential to affect how an individual responds to symptoms of a mental illness in one's self or others. Does one seek care or not? Does one seek support or not? I was one of those who did not seek care or support; but I was one of the lucky ones who used religion and it has worked thus far. Religion does not work for everyone. For this reason it is important to understand generally held beliefs about mental illness and to examine how these beliefs affect how individuals might cope with mental health problems. I know how Blacks perceived persons hospitalized for mental illness as different and inferior to normal people and believed these patients should be "restricted" to protect society. Many people in the African American community still believe depression is a personal weakness, and it is associated with shame and embarrassment and both the affected individual and the family were assumed to have the illness.

I was not ashamed nor was I embarrassed about the pain of losing my children. However, I have grieved their untimely deaths, mentally and physically. I developed GERD, high blood pressure, and other illnesses. I know that stigma associated with seeking help for mental depression kept me from seeking treatment but I am wiser now and may very well seek the help that I have so desperately needed all these years.

I was once concerned about my image. But I now understand how images and ideologies play such a pivotal role in culture. Images on the one hand, are to recognize that they are produced within the dynamics of social power and ideology; while ideologies are systems of belief that exist within all cultures. I held onto the propaganda of false representations that compromised my own interests. It was a pervasive, mundane process that I was engaged in but completely unaware of. Further, ideology is also an indispensable set of values and beliefs through which I had lived out my complex relations in a range of social structures during and after the death of my children and husband. For instance, I held on to the belief that individuals who had a mental illness within the Black community were not normal and they were harmful to themselves and to others. The image of a person with mental illness was that of a "crazy" person who should be locked up and frankly removed from society. These images kept me from seeking help for mental depression. When someone made a remark about how well I was doing under the circumstances, I always smiled but deep down inside I was coming apart.

What I did not know was the vast number of individuals in my community who had a diagnosed mental illness. And millions more, like me, may be affected but are undiagnosed. In fact, I believe women may be over-represented in the area of mental depression based on their sheer social structure, which may include their sociopolitical experiences including racism, discrimination, and sexism which put African American women at risk for low-income jobs, multiple role strain and health problems, all of which could cause an onset of mental illness. Older African American women may be at a higher risk of developing mental illness due to disability from chronic medical conditions, caregiver strain, social isolation, bereavement, exposure to traumatic events (elder abuse, violence, living in crime-ridden neighborhoods), and poor access to health care (Arean & Reynolds, 2005; Artinian, Washington, Flack, Hockman, & Jen, 2006).

Older African American women are often isolated, and sometimes isolation will also cause them to become physically ill. If it is chronic, they are at higher risk of developing mental illness. I have found that some older African American women within my ministerial circle who are living alone are suffering with some sort of illness and sometimes they forget to take their medicine or they've been known to over-medicate themselves. Forgetfulness is often associated with mental illness but the women with whom I have had first-hand experience are in denial about their condition. They will not seek professional help because of stigma. In my case, I used religion but I would have been better served if I had sought professional help. I would have been able to handle the deaths of my children and my husband. Perhaps by now I would have stopped crying.

I have not stopped crying because I realize that the loss of my children has caused me to look at other facets of my life that have disturbed my psyche all of my life. It goes back to being a child, not understanding why my skin tone was darker than my older siblings. I guess I was around seven years old when I realized that I had a different father than my nine sisters and brothers who had what is considered a fairer skin tone. I looked at my mother and her skin was a ruddy reddish Indian color (her mother was full blooded Mohican Indian) and she had long coarse hair, but my daddy's skin was dark like mine. I didn't care; I wanted to look like the rest of my family. I was dark skinned but my hair was a mixed bag of long thin hair. Beauticians always commented that my hair was half nappy and half straight. Well, as far as I was concerned, it was all nappy! Beauticians were always straightening it with a hot straightening comb and always burning my doggone ear. Where was the straight part, I wondered? So here I was, "a black skinny, nappy-haired pickaninny" as I was sometimes referred to, in a house that had been filled with sisters and brothers who were referred to as "light skinned or high yellow" with beautiful, thick somewhat wavy hair. Thank God most of them were married and living in other parts of the U.S. by the time I was born. I grew up with one brother and one sister until my sister got married at fourteen years of age (yes, you heard me right, fourteen years old), and my brother went into the military after graduating from high school. That was fine by me because I hated being the only "dark skinned" child that my mother had. When I was younger I wanted to look just like her (Indian tone –like her Mohican mother with the long thick hair). As I grew older, I began to look more and more like her, minus the skin color and long thick hair. Of course, my mother often said that I was crazy when I was younger because every time she spanked me, I accused her of spanking me because I was "black." I grew up with an unbelievable self-identity problem because of my skin color. I did not accept my skin tone until James Brown came out with the song, "Say it Loud, I'm Black and I'm Proud." I have since come to grips with my skin tone and who I am, but I did not always feel this way.

There are a lot of African American women who grew up with the same stigma. That is why they began bleaching their skin. Now they are going to the extreme by bleaching their skin and buying long straight hair because they think that it is sexy.

Yes, I wear a hair weave! My hair began to thin out because of mental depression.

I was like many African American women when it came to identifying that I had a mental health issue dating back to my childhood. I did not attribute my inability to sleep at night or my stoic existence to a mental imbalance. It took me a decade to come to grips with the fact that I was suffering from mental depression and some additional years to let the words come from my mouth. When I could say, "I was mentally depressed," that was the day the tears dried up. I was not ashamed nor was I embarrassed about the pain of losing my entire family. I just did not know how to cope with my losses. But I have come to realize that prayer really changes things. I was hanging by a thread in the abyss when God rescued me. I have grieved my children's untimely deaths both mentally and physically. My mental state and my physical body were breaking down simultaneously because I developed GERD, high blood pressure, and other illnesses. I know that stigma associated with seeking help for mental depression kept me from seeking treatment but I am wiser now and may very well seek the help that I have so desperately needed. Likewise, I will encourage other women from all walks of life to seek help for mental stresses in their lives, to stop letting stigmas bind them up. Now that I know better, I will do better. I will speak truth to power so that others might know that it is possible to get help where help is needed. I will bring mental health care professionals into the church and bring the community together so they will know that the stigmas that have kept them bound are just that—a stigma. I will seek to educate and eradicate the feelings of alienation when African American women are faced with mental health issues.

There is power in knowledge and I will seek to empower African American women by providing knowledge about mental health treatments. I will not make a joke about such a serious illness. When I said to God, "You have got to be joking," I meant it. But God does not joke when He has a job for us to do.

GOD'S GOT JOKES

It really seemed like a cruel joke for God to show me visions when I had not fully grieved the loss of my children. Nevertheless, God "called" me in the midst of my pain and suffering and I answered with some hesitation, "Here am I, send me" after questioning God about waking me up every morning at 3:30 am.

I was "called" by God but I have endured unusual roadblocks. One would think dying to live would be smooth sailing since it was a call from God. Not so; the road back has been nothing short of a slippery treacherous slope and should have hindered my capacity to honor God's call. But I have persevered because I am aware of who I am and who "called" me. I know my true self. As a female pastor of one of the leading denominations in the world I have faced many challenges which tested my authenticity and moral compass. First, there is the familiar sexist double standard; I faced the paradox of constructing myself as a leader in a male dominated culture. Webster defines culture as, "the integrated pattern of human knowledge, belief, and behavior that depends upon the capacity for learning and transmitting knowledge to succeeding generations." Therefore, the culture of the religious community's belief systems, etc., is inherently male-oriented. If the norms for the workplace and leadership are both stereotypically masculine, women are less likely to be perceived as potential leaders, and those who do move into leadership face a double bind between being professional and being feminine. Some men have even questioned why I was appointed to the United Methodist Church that I now serve. They were under the impression that it was a full-time appointment until I opened my big mouth and told them that it was not.

Secondly, I faced the problem of performing as an associate pastor in an all-white church and as a senior pastor of an all-Black church, roles which have arguably been male dominated roles. I was the first African American female associate pastor in the white church and the first female pastor in the 138 year history of the Black church that I currently serve. This is complicated further by both settings being religious settings in communities of practice that value their cultural norms and in which each cultural norm is different.

I was hired as an associate pastor in an all-White church shortly after abandoning the all-Black church. I was licensed and ordained in a Black Baptist church and it is where my original pastoral identity was constructed. It was the place where I performed religiously as a scripture reader and altar-call prayer leader. According to Melina (2013), performances and performative discourses reveal cultural meanings, some of which are invisible except as expressed through embodied culture. A female minister reading scripture and praying reveal imbedded cultural meanings of which I was not aware. This was acceptable behavior for a female associate pastor in a Baptist church (Black or White).

I knew coming into the ministry that I could not expect much, when I told my pastor I had been "called." But God has got a way of making His vision plain, and He did it through my now deceased husband. Through my husband's emergency heart surgery, God moved not only on his behalf but also on my behalf. My husband almost died on the operating table and seven and one half hours later his doctor came to me to tell me to pray if I had a relationship with God. I did not pray right away, but I began to cry and I began to look for the prayer warrior from the church but she could not be found. I was forced to pray. I did not ask my pastor to pray; I prayed as the doctor had instructed. When I stopped praying I knew that my husband would be fine and I said as much to my pastor. Not only would he be fine but so would I because when I stopped praying my pastor looked at me with a new respect in his eyes and said, "If I didn't know that you were 'called' before, I know it now and as soon as you are able to return to the church you will be placed under 'Watch-care.'" I was licensed in 1994 and served as an Associate Pastor from 1994 through 2001. And while I was ordained during this time (1997) and went on to earn a Master of Divinity Degree in 2001, nothing changed at the Baptist church. It was just a formality as far as they were concerned. I remained an Associate Pastor and a member of the pastoral team with no additional responsibilities until God moved me to a denomination that was more open to female pastors. As I reflect on the events of my life before and after God Called me to take up my cross and follow Him, I can now see how God's plans for me and my ministerial journey has unfolded. I initially joined an all-Black United Methodist church but was subsequently hired as an associate pastor in an all-White church within the denomination.

THE DELIVERY ROOM

ALTHOUGH I WAS hired to jump-start the emerging church, I also preached in the traditional church once a month. I performed my duties as the lead preacher in the emerging church and the traditional church as requested, notwithstanding the fact that I was the first female and first African American male or female to grace either pulpit. Candace West (1977) makes the claim that if the ground of gender identity is the stylized repetition of acts through time, and not a seemingly seamless identity, then the possibilities of gender transformation are to be found in the arbitrary relations between such acts, in the possibility of a different sort of repeating, in the breaking or subversive repletion of the style. In fact, I performed my acts so well, I was able to generate a "call and response" from the all-White church that I had declared was spiritually dead because they sat there not emitting any emotions, so I thought. I did not see the tears that flowed from the eyes of the women (young and old) therefore I could not believe the response to the call. I had to ask my prayer partner, Connie Jacobus, if I had heard correctly. When she looked up at me with a big grin and said, "Every one of them," I knew that I had turned the corner wherein my race and gender did not matter. Butler (1988) argues that if gender is instituted through acts which are internally discontinuous then the appearance of substance is precisely that, a constructed identity, a performative accomplishment which the mundane social audience, including the actor themselves, comes to believe and to perform in the mode of belief. Butler (1988) further argues that if the gender identity is the stylized repetition of acts through time, and not a seemingly seamless identity, then the possibilities of gender transformation are to be found in the arbitrary relation between such acts, in the possibility of a different sort of repeating, in the breaking or subversive repetition of that style.

As the congregation came to know me, what started out as a performative accomplishment soon changed as my identity changed. The rituals of communion, baptism, weddings, and funerals changed my constructed identity. The aspects of performativity drew me into a sacred place where there was neither male nor female.

My narrative identity changed as I became their pastor--not just an African American female associate hired to jump-start the emerging church but an authentic pastor. My salary remained the same because, after all, I could not make more than the White male associate even though promises had been made. But it did not matter, because God moved and my status changed in the eyes of the congregants. I began to embody what it meant to pastor individuals from another culture and as a result they began constituting my identity. The women (and some of the men) in particular, began to believe in me even though I embodied certain cultural historical possibilities, a complicated process of appropriation which any phenomenological theory of embodiment needs to describe. In order to describe the gendered body, a phenomenological theory of constitution requires an expansion of the conventional view of acts to mean both that which constitutes meaning and that through which meaning is performed or enacted. In other words, the acts by which gender is constituted bear similarities to performative acts within theatrical contexts. Jackson (2004) gives credence to this argument by adding that, agency lies in the work of performativity. Because subjects are constantly reproduced (through repetition), they are never fully constituted. There is always space for reworking and resisting. And because subjects can subversively transform, refuse, parody, or rupture the laws of discourse, thereby reconstituting themselves, identities emerge from discourse and power relations as neither foundational grounds nor fully expressed products. Jackson (2004) very eloquently grapples with the discourses of the historical processes that constitute who one is, and the location and nature of power relations inherent in them, which make possible the *self-knowledge* that she constructs about oneself and the "wording" of their world. This type of grappling helps the writer remember buried treasures of her early life as a female minister, one being the revitalization of the women's Bible study group at the all-White southern church. The women were thirsty for an interactive Bible study and wanted to act outside of the norms. They wanted to deconstruct in order to find a construct suitable to who they really were--not who someone else said they were. De Lauretis (1984) argued that the process of constructing subjectivity is an important concern for feminists because subjectivity is produced by a woman's "personal, subjective engagement in the practices, discourses, and institutions that lend significance (value, meaning, and affect) to the events of the world." Weedon (1997) called for a poststructural feminism that attends to situated meaning as an effect of language. "The meaning of the signifier 'woman' varies from the ideal to victim to object of sexual desire, according to its context. The context for the forty-seven women was as self-defining for them as it was for me. Within this context, I found the courage to tell my story. By telling my story through the biblical text, the forty-seven were liberated and found the courage to tell their stories. The narratives that were shared were (re)presentations of episodes in their construction of subjectivity as White southern women to provide "data" that illuminates. The women trusted me and one another intimately because I became their authentic leader, worthy of carrying and storing the burdens of their pain in my heart as they did mine.

Nearly fifteen years after my departure from this church and unparalleled Bible Study group, we are still near and dear to one another because of our shared experiences.

MY AUTHENTIC SELF

GENERALLY, AUTHENTICITY IS defined in leadership literatures as absence of self-deception, recognition of any shortcomings, striving for the fulfillments of individual potential, having self-awareness of purpose, taking full responsibility for one's error, and being one's true self (Shamir & Eilam, 2005, Sparrowe, 2005; Avolio & Gardner, 2005; Ilies, Morgeson & Nahrgang, 2005). Within this context, authenticity as an inner individual moral self-concept can be observed and influence positive behaviors as leaders and the action of leadership. This notion is also supported by Chan, Hannah, and Gardner (2005) from a social cognitive lens. They suggested that authenticity has two features: (1) the presence and awareness of a core self with the self-system; and (2) presentation of self to align with core self. Through a psychological lens, Kernis (2003) asserted that authenticity can be characterized as reflecting the unobstructed operation of one's true or core self. Avolio and Gardner (2005), from a moral perspective, asserted that leaders are described authentic if they undergo rigorous self-reflection to understand their moral compasses, and engage in practices appropriate to inner self-perception. Female ministers have had to navigate some very treacherous situations in order to be recognized as leaders. If one does not have a good understanding of one's true self, and if they have not undergone rigorous self-reflection in order to understand their moral compass and call to ministry, they cannot withstand the test of time.

According to Opatokun, Hasim, and Hasan, (2013), this is the phenomenon most required by institutions of higher learning due to their roles in nation-building and human capacity development. Most prior studies on authentic leadership focused on specific contexts and sectors such as the top executives and CEOs of corporate organizations (George, Sim, McLean, and Mayer, 2007); auditors' behavior (Morris, 2010); corporate organization (Roux, 2010; Walumbwa, Avolio, Gardner, Wernsing, & Peterson, 2008) and military leadership (Beyer, 2010). Despite these widespread acknowledgements of the importance of authentic leadership as an emerging theory in education, there is little empirical evidence. Against this backdrop, the purpose of this book is to tell the story of how I had to die in order to live but it is also to test my self-awareness, balanced processing of information, internalized moral perspective, and relational transparency as predictors of authentic leadership among female ministers.

The new leadership paradigm requires leaders with a stable philosophical and psychological self for the continuity of the organization as a social system. My philosophical self was pretty much intact but that is where it ended. And here is the dilemma; my psychological self was in tatters when I was hired to jumpstart the Emerging Church. Arguably researchers and/or practitioners are of the opinion that, with the development and study of authentic leaders, leaders' preferential interests are overtly taken by self-awareness, self-regulations, positive modeling, ethical reasoning, relational transparency, and balanced processing. They lead through a solid understanding of their moral, ethical and inner self, with greater self-awareness and self-regulation of positive behaviors in themselves and those that they lead (Luthans & Avolio, 2003). In addition, authentic leadership is considered (Avolio & Gardner, 2005; Begley, 2003; Walumbwa et al., 2008; George, 2003) to be particularly important in achieving organizational objectives, and in evolving effectiveness among subordinates. Also, authentic leaders might be a congregation's saving grace from the shackles of leaders who have their personal interest at heart before considering others. By professing positive images, the preferential interests of leaders are blindsided, submerged, and buried by the needs of groups, organization, community, and culture. If not (Begley, 2003), they joined the congregation of failed leaders. While all this may seem to constitute positive attributes of authentic leaders, understandingly there is a deliberating question against authentic leadership, study and development that poses challenges: how do individuals shun preferential interest for the collective interest of the organization? Secondly, how do leaders reconcile their preferential interests with those of the organization? Consequently, there might be a mismatch between individual personality and organizational roles when leaders compromise their values, integrity, identity, images, and morality by acting against their moral consciousness.

FIRST FEMALE

THE ALL-BLACK CHURCH where I continue to pastor is quite a paradigm shift from the role that I had previously held at the all-White church. However, I came with an open heart ready to love the people, knowing that I had to earn their trust as I had done at the previous church. I also knew that people had to see that I was an authentic leader through my life story. I knew that authentic leadership rests heavily on the self-relevant meanings that leaders attach to their life experiences, and these experiences are captured in the leader's life stories. I also knew that the Black church is much like the Black barber shop, except there is no fading, twisting and weaving. And, I knew that it is a cultural site for ethnographic exploration and description (Alexander, 2003). It is also a constructed community for spiritual, social and intellectual discourse. Leda M. Cook (1998) states that, "cultural spaces are infused with the past, markers of identity that are creative and created through historical events and experiences." A cultural space is a particular site marked by the cultural practices of the people who live there (or lived there in the case of ritual burial grounds and battlefields). According to Alexander (2003), these spaces serve as a register of cultural identity denoting but not delimiting bodies distinguished by race, practices, and styles of cultural membership.

The Black church that I currently serve was organized more than 151 years ago and has all of the trappings of an authentic cultural space with burial grounds and many of the cultural practices inherent to Black people. It is a contemporary church with up tempo music accompanied by an organ player and drummer, and from time to time, bass and lead guitars. The pastor is expected to lead a worship service that complements a contemporary church setting. His or her performance becomes necessary for the survival of the church. Religious services are considered cultural performance, according to Conquergood (1998). Self-conscious and symbolic acts are presented and communicated within a circumscribed space. Meaning and affect are generated by embodied action that produces a heightened moment of communication.

Cultural performance inheres to what the ethnolinguistic Richard Bauman (1977) calls "markings." It is framed by its content both within and outside the flow of life as lived, as well as by its distinct markings of beginnings and endings (Bauman, 1977). According to Conquergood (1982), you cannot stumble into a cultural performance and be oblivious to it.

If it is true that cultural performances are not only a reflection of what we are, they also shape and direct who we are and what we can become (Turner, 1982a), I stand in anticipation of what is in store as I continue on the journey that I am on in this performance called life. On this journey I am an authentic spiritual leader ready to lead God's people into the "promised land." I came as Moses did with all of my weaknesses.

I am reminded that in addition to the leader presenting the self as an authentic leader, the church has a responsibility to the leader as well. The denomination finally lived up to its promise to transfer my ordination in 2017. It is too late! I keep reflecting on this elder who was supposed to be mentoring me, but had made up in her mind when she met me, that I would never be a Methodist. She said at our first meeting, "But, you will not.' All of these Baptist's coming in here wanting to be Methodist." " Well guess what, I am! And, I have served the Methodist church honorably for nearly 19 years; 15 of which as senior pastor.

And just as she called it, my credentials were never transferred because she demonized me in front of a cadre of elders who had to vote on the transference. She may have stopped them, but she could not stop God and I am still serving in the Methodist church and I am reappointed each year (currently into my 14th year) as a Retired Licensed Local UMC Pastor. What this woman meant for evil God meant it for my good because several years after that dreadful experience, I went back to school to earn a Ph.D. in interdisciplinary studies with a concentration in leadership. And, God has raised me up in the church in spite of her viciousness. I was appointed as the leader over seven other churches while holding on to my identity as a pastor from another denomination, and I currently serve on the Atlanta Decatur Oxford Disrict's Trustee/Finance Committe.

When I was first appointed to the church I was told that the church was not "ready" for a female pastor. The church was not ready for a female pastor, but a female was ready to pastor the church. I was ready to pastor because along the way, I began to construct my personal identity based on the roads that I had already traveled. My narrative identity was already established. I was a rebel whom God had called to pastor His church in this present age. Therefore, this narrative approach to my "tedious journey" is a way of focusing on the stories in which I am able to construct through my personal and social identities. I have narratives that constitute multiple identities and the stories of life shape my narrative identities. My narratives have a long history of tedious journeys. It has taken me to the pits of hell but I have come out stronger than before. It has taken me from the role of a civil rights activist, to corporate meeting rooms, to entrepreneurship, to numerous struggles with the "Death Angel," to the halls of a seminary, to the pulpit, to the university halls, to boardrooms. Each of these narratives and their relationship to each other are transformative. My social identity in the Northeast is recognizable as the leader of a local and state civil rights organization. In the Southeast, I am recognized as a Methodist pastor, a seminary professor, a director of a mentoring program, a charter school governance board member chairing teaching and learning, A GED founder and director, and a substitute school teacher. In all of this, my way back from the abyss has been debilitating. In each of these groups I am a recognized member and I perform the roles required of each group though it has not been without a struggle.

Even though I had struggles as a seminary professor, I found healing in the midst of the chaos. I was hired as a seminary adjunct professor immediately after I earned the Doctor of Ministry degree. When the director of ministry and context called to offer me a position on his staff in July 2003, I could not believe my good fortune. I had just graduated in May, so I thought to myself "God is really not a joke." Of course, I readily accepted the offer. And after attending a few meetings so that I would understand all that the position entailed, I stood in front of my first group of students scared to death at the beginning of the fall 2003 semester. God had given me the platform that I said I did not have when I was first called into ministry. I could tell my students that Jesus loved them, and not only that, I could demonstrate Jesus' love to those who had acknowledged their call and entered seminary, not knowing how they would eat, sleep or have the basic necessities of life.

I was in for a rude awakening about seminary life and the sacrifices that so many students made when they responded to the call. When I entered seminary I came bearing the burden of my losses. Few if any of my students were grieving the loss of entire families, but they came under heavy burdens of illnesses, i.e., cancer, HIV/AIDS, loss of spouses to same gender relationships, strokes, heart disease and the list goes on. It was my job to train the students to use their burdens as a catalyst to share the goodness and love of Jesus Christ to those who needed to hear from God through Word and Deed. In spite of what they were going through, God was waiting on them, for surely they had been called and set apart. Being in the seminary setting gave new meaning to Luke 4:18-19 when Jesus declared, "The Spirit of the Lord is upon me..." It became clearer to me how God uses our brokenness to help others who so desperately need to hear from God. God used the seminarians to preach good news to the poor, to heal the brokenhearted, to give sight to the blind, and to set the captives free. They came with all of their baggage, sometimes with no place to lay their heads, with empty stomachs, and not a dime in their pockets until student loans were dispersed. But they had come to learn how to do the will of He who sent them.

God set me in places of leadership, not to look down upon the students, but to look after them in their hour of need. When I learned that they were hungry, my class opened the first food pantry pretty much at the expense of the writer because most of the students lived a meager existence. We sought help from the institution but it was taking too long. The students needed immediate help and several of us made it a priority. When rent was due and the students had no money, we reached out to in-house organizations for help. And in some instances some relief was made available, but in most cases there was dead silence. In times like these, God always made a way out of no way.

The same type of things happened when the writer was promoted to the director's position for a mentoring program for 1st year seminarians and post graduates. There was the brokenness but not the poverty because they received a monthly stipend. In an effort to help students see the need to stay in the church we provided workshops and mentors to encourage them along the way. I loved directing this program because we saw God in action. God's presence was seen and felt all over the place through what we did and what we experienced.

The mentoring program gave me another audience and another opportunity for God to show me that He was not joking when he called me to tell His people that He loved them. Everything that I did and everything that I said had the love of God all over it. From the places that we stayed, the food that we ate, the workshops that we attended, and the open sessions that we gathered in, God's love abounded. God showed up in the testimonies, the sermons, the songs that we sang, and in the gathering of the sheep. If I had any doubt about God's ability to use me in his glory, it soon disappeared. God knows how to use a rebel! Rebels learn quickly that God is not a joke. If I learned nothing else from teaching and directing programs at the seminary, I learned that you just don't tell God that He has to be joking, nor do you tell God that you have no way of carrying out His mandates. Through these two experiences alone, God allowed me to tell hundreds of people that He loved them. It seemed like an insurmountable task when God called me but God gave the audiences to me in increments. And the beauty of it was, God had even more for me to do at the seminary. I chaired several conferences and fundraisers for various departments. The work that I did widened my territory and audiences even more. In the process, I learned to let the Holy Spirit lead and guide me to all understanding.

This experience was just another narrative that was scripted by God.

In the many different disciplines in which narratives have been studied, organizational management researchers have placed considerable emphasis on the importance of stories for their role on myth and sense-making in organizations (Boje, 1991; Dennehy, 1999; Fleming, 2001; Kaye, 1996; Ready, 2002). Frequently the focus of these researchers has been the way stories communicate important information.

My personal identity has never changed. I am the same in the Southeast as I was in the Northeast. I constructed my sameness. Rebels have a way of constructing themselves with sameness. It was no easy task because there have been so many roadblocks, Also, I have had so many conflicting social identities out of which I have had to weave my personal identity.

It may seem farfetched, but I have had to create and re-create my personal identity out of memories of events in my own life and the lives of my now deceased family. This undertaking is a way of trying to make sense of a rebel's life by unifying my experiences, scripts, and social identities and projecting them into the future; and it is not easy.

As I reflect on my journey from the abyss and the margins (struggles on the streets of Connecticut as a civil rights leader) to the pulpit, I have vivid memories of board of education meetings where I along with others, challenged the board as they sought to close all inner city schools (one is still standing). And now I find myself challenging DeKalb County officials about a landfill in my church community. Rebels do not accept the status quo. God will not allow it. Standing boldly, my social identity as a civil rights leader was projected into the future, and here I stand integrating all of the scripts.

I am able to integrate all of the scripts because each step of the way, I have been operating out of a sense of desperation brought on by Storm Death appearing in my life for nearly two decades. Even so, I still had a determination to do the best job possible. In every struggle along the way, I have had self-determination to accomplish the goals set before me. There are those in the church who comment on my tenacity even in the face of adversity. They say things like, "I don't know how you do it." I know how I do it! It is by God's grace. When I am told no, I keep pressing the issue. If I was not a rebel, I would not have the inner strength to persevere, and I would have left the ministry a long time ago.

I was not given complete authority in the development of the emerging church as promised, and although I was treated unfairly about my pay scale, I never lost sight of who I was or what I was called to do. My dislike of how I was treated was never reflected in my actions in revamping the women's Bible study. Despite the fact that throughout this ministry journey I have remained transparent (unlike some of my male counterparts) I have not fared as well as some of the male pastors sharing the same credentials. They are appointed to the biggest and best churches in the best locations; and of course they receive the highest salaries because they have more members. These pastors hardly ever visit the sick and shut-ins and do not have outreach ministries; if they do, their faces are never seen, but "still they rise." Their followers love them and shower gifts on them while I struggle to get a birthday card. I wonder sometimes if I am too transparent with my followers.

Another issue among male pastors has to do with immorality and unethical behavior. It is worth noting that there are contentious arguments among researchers whether to include or exclude a moral component from the construct of authentic leadership. Although Luthans and Avolio (2003) conceptualize that authentic leadership and its development includes an inherent ethical/moral component, Gardner et al. (2005a), and Avolio and Gardner (2005) asserted that the construct of authentic leadership needs a positive moral/ethical component. It is contended that authentic leaders are moral agents that have high moral standards and capacities to judge moral dilemmas. They are, however, of the view that positive moral perspective is crucial to the emerging work on authentic leadership development. Other researchers (e.g., Cooper et al, 2005; Shamir & Eilam, 2005, Sparrowe, 2005) argue against the construct having a moral component, stressing that it dilutes the construct. Furthermore, Cooper et al. (2005) suggest that studies on authentic leadership are better predicated on consensus regarding theoretical frameworks and investigative methods. It is hard to believe but too many male pastors are immoral and unethical. This statement is based on the number of prominent ministers who are caught up in sex scandals wherein the church is ultimately sued. We very seldom hear of women who are caught up in sex or other scandals in the church. But then again, we do not have that many leading mainline denominational churches. As for me, my personal construct as a minister does not allow for immorality or unethical behavior.

While emphasis was also placed on the notion that knowledge cannot be advanced in a cumulative manner without reaching consensus. Cooper's study further established the view that lack of consensus in prior research (e.g. leader member exchange) leads to the replicate of efforts to create the measure of a single phenomenon. And then the research resulting from these various measures were not directly comparable. The authors concur further that authentic leadership scholars need to give careful consideration to the four critical issues: defining and measuring the construct, determining the discriminant validity of the construct, identifying relevant construct outcomes (i.e., testing the construct's nomological network), and ascertaining whether authentic leadership can be taught. In an attempt to conceptualize what constitutes authentic leadership constructs. Cooper et al. (2005) outlined research issues that formed the origin of Walumbwa et al's (2008) authentic leadership definition, measurement, and validity that is "to lay the necessary conceptual and empirical groundwork for advancing authentic leadership theory and development.

Furthermore, Walumbwa et al's (2008) authentic leadership construct conceptualization is predicated on research by Avolio and Gardner (2005), Garner et al (2005a), and Ilies et al (2005) for three reasons: (1) it is firmly rooted in the extant social psychological theory and research; (2) it explicitly recognizes and articulates the central role of internalized moral perspective to authentic leadership and its development, and (3) it focuses explicitly on the development of authentic leaders and authentic followers. They developed the following definition of authentic leadership through the modification of Luthans and Avolio's (2003) definition to advance a refined definition that reflects the underlying dimension of the Gardner et al. (2005a) and Ilies et al. (2005) constructs:

> ...as a pattern of leader behavior that draws upon and promotes both positive psychological capacities and a positive ethical climate, to foster greater self-awareness,

> and internalized moral perspective, balanced processing of information, and relational transparency on the part of leaders working with followers, fostering self-development (Walumbwa et al., 2008, p. 94).

Walumbwa et al. (2008) viewed authentic leadership as being composed of five distinct and substantive components, which are self-awareness, relational transparency, internalized regulations (i.e., authentic behavior), balanced processing of information, and positive moral perspective. The internalized regulation processes and authentic behavior were further combined into a single concept (internalized moral perspective), because the two concepts were conceptually equivalent (both involve exhibiting behaviors) from a self-determination theory perspective. As explained by Walumbwa et al. (2008), in an attempt to operationalize the authentic leadership construct, there are conceptual overlaps between the internalized regulation and positive moral perspective dimensions. Additionally, these dimensions were collapsed into a single dimension—internalized moral perspective, which involves a leader's inner drive to achieve behavioral integrity. The four constructs of authentic leadership, as identified by Walumbwa's research, formed the basis of this research. It might be safely stated at this end that the study on authentic leadership may continue to be a subject of discourse among researchers for a very long time.

And while this may be so, as we continue the discourse, we must be mindful of the four components of authentic leadership mentioned earlier in this paper, the first of which is self-awareness. The notion is that self-awareness is a central element in authentic leadership study, with an interest on identifying how self-awareness can be perceived in leaders' behaviors. According to Klenke (2005), self-awareness is the degree to which an individual is aware of various aspects of self-identities, and congruent with the ways they are perceived by others. Self-awareness then is a measure of the ability to be truly conscious of self-components and to observe it without prejudice. The majority of literature on self-awareness suggests that it involves awareness of, and trust in, individual personal characteristics, values, motives, feelings, and cognition.

Walking into an all-White church and meeting with an all-White Board tells me that I am truly conscious of my self-components. I had no knowledge of how I would be received and had not met any of the interviewing body. But I went in with the confidence of being aware of who I was and what I could bring to the church. And it worked out for me and for them. I left the women in a better place than they were when I arrived and the men began to better understand race and gender.

I did not know what to expect when I walked into the pulpit of the all-Black United Methodist church as their pastor. But I walked in under the authority of the Holy Spirit, knowing that God had called me for such a time as this. Having a Black female pastor was a first for the church and my first as the lead pastor of any church.

Relational transparency is the next component and it is found in Kernis' (2003) research, which was referred to as relational authenticity. Relational authenticity involves endorsing the importance for others to see the real you, either good or bad. I strive to enable individuals to see the real me. It is important to develop relational authenticity, particularly in a church environment. I believe that I accomplished that goal in both church settings because of the personal invitations that I received to be involved in family events. You are not welcome at the table unless there is an authentic relationship. Authentic leaders are transparent in expressing their true emotions and feelings (Gardner et al 2005a). Concurrently they regulate such emotions to reduce display of inappropriate emotions. By responding transparently to moral dilemmas, authentic leaders become ethical role models (Gardner & Schermerhorn, 2004). Nevertheless, Hughes (2005) argues that relational transparency results from the leaders' self-disclosure which is comprised of four aspects: goals/motives, identity, values and emotions (GIVE). The leader is transparent to the followers when making ethical decisions and, to be transparent, one must be self-aware of one's weaknesses and strengths.

Internalized moral perspective is an essential moral consideration which is at the very heart of the leadership relationship. Recent leadership literature recognized the growing meditation in value and taking value positions. I believe that I have consistently demonstrated what it means to internalize a moral perspective in all of my leadership endeavors. It would have been impossible to be an authentic leader without a moral compass and a commitment to transparency. The degree of commitment of the organization's leader to ethical conduct and values are very important and thus influence the followers and the organization in a positive way. Walumbwa et al. (2008) are of the notion that self-regulation is "guided by internal moral standards and values versus group, organizational, and societal pressures, and it results in expressed decision making and behavior that is consistent with these internalized values. Leaders exhibit ethical behaviors when they are doing what is morally right, just, and good. When they do so, they help elevate followers' awareness and moral self-actualization. This has always been my goal. I want followers to see the good in me even when I am being treated unfairly. Even if they do not follow my example, at least they know that this is one pastor who tried to do the right thing.

COPING WITH MENTAL DEPRESSION

FINALLY, THE BALANCED processing of information can be comprehended by taking into consideration how motivational biases impact the processes by which people with low or fragile high esteem opt for and understand information. The point of argument is that there is need for frameworks and ways of thinking that will encompass the full range of human motivation and valuation processes as it relates to leadership practices and serves as a guide to action, particularly as a support to ethical resolution of dilemmas. Ethics and moral and valuation models are important for institutional leadership to serve as rubrics, benchmarks, social standards of practice, and templates for moral actions. To serve as a template for moral actions, balanced processing refers to the impartial collection of relevant self-related information, either positive or negative in nature. That is, the leader does not distort, exaggerate, or ignore externally based evaluations of the self nor internal experiences and private knowledge that might inform self-development (Gardner et al., 2005a). Balanced processing of information involves being aware of and attuned to one's weaknesses and strengths, and care is taken to deflect from the weakness angle when needs call for it. Balanced processing refers to leaders who show that they objectively scrutinize all pertinent information before making any conclusions the reported 2.1 gender ratio of depression. Additionally sociopolitical experiences including racism, discrimination, and sexism put African American women at risk for low-income jobs, multiple role strain and health problems, all of which are associated with the onset of mental illness. Older African American women may be at a higher risk of developing mental illness due to disability from chronic medical conditions, caregiver strain, social isolation, bereavement, exposure to traumatic events (elder abuse, violence, living in crime-ridden neighborhoods), and poor access to health care.

Older African American women are often isolated, and sometimes isolation will also cause them to become physically ill. If it is chronic, they are at higher risk of developing mental illness. It has been my experience that most older women are suffering with some sort of illness and sometimes they forget to take their medicine or have been known to over-medicate themselves. Forgetfulness is often associated with mental illness. But because of stigma, they will not seek professional help.

I have been in need of a psychological support system for many years. Instead, I sought healing through God. I cried and I prayed but I would not seek professional help even if I knew psychologists because individuals in the community would have said that

I could not cope, that I'd had a nervous breakdown; and I was determined not to let it happen. The rebel in me would not let go. I did not know that crying at the mention of my children was a crippling mental disorder. It was nothing to be ashamed of but I told myself that as a civil rights leader I had to be strong. After all, I had an image to maintain. I had to handle myself correctly. Neighbors, Musick and Williams (1998) found that cultural beliefs appear to affect coping behaviors. There are certain common patterns that can be found in the African American community. However, coping with mental illness without treatment is not necessarily an African American female problem or civil rights leader's issue. Studies (Owen, 2003) have shown that mental illnesses amongst politicians are often difficult to diagnose and, even if diagnosed, it may be impossible to ensure treatment. For instance, the Ugandan President Idi Amin was responsible for random killings and appalling abuses of human rights. Questions were raised about his mental state. But the state of his mental health, just as for many other leaders, was never substantiated, and perhaps never will be. Who would have thought that President Reagan was unfit mentally to be president of the United States? His battery of tests included having to subtract 7 from 10. Then there was President John F. Kennedy who suffered from Addison's disease and was treated with steroids. Had it been known, he never would have beaten Richard Nixon in a very tight race in 1960. My point is, civil rights leaders as well as politicians have images to maintain and have to often cover up medical histories. But the stress and anxiety of maintaining an image, reinforced by the cultural community, can have deleterious effects on coping behaviors and health (Neal-Barnett & Crowther, 2000), such as in the case of the cultural stereotype of the strong Black woman. While I was crumbling inside, I continued to believe that I had an image to maintain; that I had to handle myself correctly; I had to be a strong Black woman. I loved it when someone commented on how strong I was. If they only knew! Maintaining the image of the self-reliant Black woman might delay or hinder treatment-seeking among African American women. Adding to the researcher's argument, I would like to point out that there are millions of African American women like myself who do not seek treatment because of the very issues that Matthews, Mays et al., found. I am in treatment now. Trauma has a way of bringing you to your knees. Neighbors, Musick, & Williams also found that African American women were more likely to seek help from ministers; if a minister was contacted first, the likelihood of seeking help from other sources was decreased. African Americans tend to rely on family and religious and social networks for emotional support rather than seek out professional care. As an African American woman and pastor, I've seen firsthand how friends and family who have gone through bouts of depression look to the church or faith community for help instead of seeking professional help. Churches are an important social community for many African Americans. A sense of connection and safety surrounds the church, and people tend to trust the church more than a health care system. Individuals in the church look to prayer for healing, but more church leaders like me are saying that prayer alone is not sufficient and that mental health services are needed. This provides an opportunity for the medical community and faith-based organization to collaborate to provide services to the African American community. I sought the prayers of my pastor initially, and then I sought God for myself. And I did handle myself in the best way that I knew how. I walked the floor at night and I lay on the couch with a pillow over my head by day. I was mentally depressed but I was in denial about my mental health. Then again, I cannot say that I was in denial. It was more like being uninformed. I felt weighed down and I knew that the feelings were a result of my family's deaths, but I could not put my finger on a clear understanding of any one particular feeling. I knew that I did not like to be around the children's friends; and I knew that I was at a loss when it came to my husband's death but I could not say definitively what the feelings were like because they fluctuated. One day in a dark hole, next day irritable. One day I want to sleep, the next day, I just didn't want to be bothered. Today I know that I was mentally depressed. But, mentally depressed or not, something had to change because I now had two little boys to care for; so I prayed and reminded God that he had given me these precious lives and I needed to be able to sleep at night so that I could care for the boys during the day. God heard my cry and I began to sleep at night but I was still an emotional wreck. Everything made me cry and I needed help to get through each day, but I did not seek it. I flat out refused antidepressants. I ended up in the hospital for four days after my husband's death and while I was there, I was given antidepressants. When I was released, I stopped taking the pills immediately. When I went to the pharmacy, I told the pharmacist not to fill the one called Elavil. I am glad that I made the decision not to fill the prescription because it's quite likely that I would still be taking the drug today. Stigma that was so pervasive in the African American community would be my constant companion if God had not rescued me. I would not advise others to do what I did because I understand that there are those who have to take medication, and there is no shame in taking it nor should there be shame in seeking psychological help. I have needed it for a very long time.

I have since learned that I am not alone; African American women are burdened down by mental illness but their use of mental health services is low (Matthew and Hughes, 2001; Neal-Barrett & Crowder, 2000). What sets me apart is the way God crafted me. God gave me a spirit of rebellion. And the Lord knew that I would need it on this journey back from the abyss. There were so many times during the journey in which I would have just thrown in the towel and let Satan have his way.

I said in the opening chapters that it was a five year journey into the abyss when in actuality it was more like a twelve year journey if I take into account the many twists and turns that my life took from my daughter's death to my husband's death. I have to account for his open heart surgery and recovery period during this time. It occurred less than a year after my oldest son's death. That was no small matter and it would have left me in limbo if we did not have some very special friends who just happened to stop by on their way home from a Florida vacation. They stayed at our home and cared for the boys while I made my daily treks back and forth to the hospital.

In spite of the twelve year sentence in the eye of "Storm Death," I persevered and never sought help as I journeyed into the abyss. I could not in all good conscience seek help because of the cultural stigma associated with mental depression. It would have almost signaled my death. I would have lost my identity as a professor, a leader, and a pastor. I could not take a chance on losing myself, so I walked around smiling when life had nearly crushed me inward. Stigma has been identified as the most significant barrier to seeking mental health services among African Americans but very little attention has been given to examining stigma, the beliefs about mental illness that may be associated with stigma, and how these beliefs may affect the approach to coping. But stigmas are real, and are arguably the most significant barrier to seeking mental health services among African Americans.

African American women's use of mental health services also may be influenced by barriers, including (inaccessible location, transracial and ethnic minority clinicians; transportation problems, lack of health insurance, and poverty), availability of services (limited access to culturally competent clinicians and case management) and cultural matching (few opportunities to work with racial and ethnic minority clinicians).Until the Affordable Health Care Plan went into effect, forty percent of African Americans reported being uninsured compared to one in four whites. Income was not a factor in the report of being uninsured; nearly a quarter of African Americans making more than $84,000 a year lacked coverage at some point, compared to 16 percent of whites in the same income bracket. Due to the lack of insurance, African Americans are more likely to use emergency care services. However, these health professionals do not have the expertise to diagnose and treat mental and behavioral health problems. For those with insurance, coverage for mental health services and substance disorders is still substantially lower than coverage for other medical illnesses, such as hypertension and diabetes.

Cristancho and colleagues created a vulnerability model that outlined the interaction of two types of barriers: (a) system-level barriers—those that are created by systems designed to provide mental health service, and (b) individual-level barriers—how individuals view and experience their encounters with the system (interpersonal and intrapersonal; Among the barriers, stigma has been identified as the most significant (DHHS, 2001) because it is both a system- and individual-level barrier. Other system-level barriers include the issues listed above plus social issues such as a lack of child care. In addition, a sociopolitical history involving trauma and victimization of African Americans served to foster cultural mistrust toward the U.S. health care system. At times it was misunderstood, ignored, or stigmatized. The rates of mental illness in the African American community are similar to those of the general population. Yet, according to the National Institute of Mental Illness, the African American community is underserved by the nation's mental health system. One out of three African Americans who need care for a mental illness receives it. Often, mental illness in the African American community can be seen as "just the blues" or "just acting crazy" and cause individuals not to seek professional treatment. Even violent behavior toward African American women is viewed as "acting crazy." In hindsight, no one "acts crazy;" the individuals have a mental disorder and could be helped if we (meaning the African American community) would stop ignoring the symptoms related to the person's mental health.

"Acting crazy," began during slavery. Slave's fear of being-in-general according to Earl (1996) required that they, in the face of their masters, repress the original creative self with which God had endowed them. This fear demanded that slaves act according to the dehumanizing specifications of slave masters' image of the ideal slave. Slaves overcame this fear only when they had been what they termed "struck dead" or "slain in the Spirit by God." Before this salvific experience the slave undoubtedly would not have been able to define the root sources of his or her fear. This experience gave slaves the critical means of seeing why they had been fearful of being-in-general. Conversion sources make it clear that slaves equated the fear of having to confront the malevolent master with confronting the devil. They expressed this fear to God during that phase of their visionary experiences when God would command them to reenter the plantation world as a moral witness. God's gift of courage gave the transformed self the sense of being radically free spiritually in the world of bondage. This pull and tug between the master and God may have caused psychological damage to the slaves; but I believe that God (the church) helps the converts to see that fear comes from within rather than the malevolent master.

The lack of courage to be in the face of psychological adversity seems to be the primary enemy of young African American females' upward mobility. It is normal to grow faint of spirit and weak of heart, but too many African American females are sacrificing themselves, The body of study of the moral lives of African American leaders such as DuBois, Washington, and King must be viewed as a prolegomenon of what needs to be done in future studies. I believe that the black community has failed when it comes to helping African American females and young African Americans in general to recover their rich history--to be courageous and stand in the face of adversities such as mental depression, etc.

African American women tend to reference emotions related to mental illness as "evil" or "acting out." Feelings of hyperirritability, negativity, stress and repetitive harmful impulses are also signs that you or someone you know has a mental disorder. They must face these feelings by seeking mental health treatment.

Caucasians experience mental health issues more often, but African American and Caribbean women experience greater severity and persistence. The National Survey of American Life: a study of racial, ethnic and cultural influences on mental disorder and mental health, provided evidence of communities holding on to long legacies of being subject to the slavemaster of mental illness. It is a moral challenge, Earl (1996) says, to help young African Americans recover the secret of courage that their ancestors once knew and displayed. Robert Franklin's instructive secrets reveal lies and shame originating from slavery. Avoiding emotions was a survival technique which has now become a cultural habit.

In 2008, 6.0 percent of African Americans age 18-25 had a serious mental illness in the past year. Overall, only 58.7 percent of Americans with serious mental illness received care within the past twelve months, and the percentage of African Americans receiving services is only 44.8 percent. Some populations within the African American community are more susceptible to mental illness and are more likely not to have access to specialty care. These individuals are more at risk for mental illness due to over-representation in homeless populations, individuals who are incarcerated, children in foster care and child welfare systems, and victims of serious violent crimes. These social determinants of health—where we live, learn, work, and grow—have significant impact on a person's health and health disparities. According to a report from the Commission to Build a Healthier America, supported by the Robert Wood Johnson Foundation, education and income have a vast impact on one's health. A national survey found that 67 percent of registered voters believed a higher educational level can have a positive influence on a person's health, and 68 percent believed lower income can have a negative influence on a person's health. Poor education and low income are linked to low-income jobs, living in unsafe neighborhoods with low-quality housing, and limited access to quality health services, which in turn can lead to homelessness, incarceration, or becoming a victim of a violent crime. This data verifies what we have consistently declared about the low-economic status of many African Americans. The results of the report by the Commission to Build a Healthier America cannot be minimized; it has a vast impact on millions of African Americans who do not have the wherewithal to "pull themselves up by the bootstraps." They cannot do it without proper jobs, safe neighborhoods, decent housing and of course affordable health care. Far too many African Americans and poor people are uninsured and are less likely to receive recommended preventive and primary care services. They face significant barriers to care, and ultimately face worse health outcomes. I supported the President's Affordable Health Care Plan. There are still too many people in the African American community who do not have health care, and as a result do not seek help for any health-related issues.

All of the issues mentioned above are pervasive in the African American communities whether they are rural, urban or suburban communities. In fact, in the early 1970s, rural individuals became more widely recognized as an underserved population despite myths regarding the superior quality of rural life. This recognition grew out of investigations of psychiatric utilization and morbidity in rural areas; these investigations continue to evolve and contribute to the understanding of rural-urban differences in mental health status problems endemic to rural mental health service delivery are attributable to social, economic, and geographic factors. Investigation of the relative contribution of these factors has been complicated by the difficulty in disentangling the effects of poverty from effects of race and social isolation associated with rural life, especially in the South. In addition, when treatment is received, the quality of care typically is suboptimal, particularly among minorities. Although this situation is discouraging, it is hardly surprising given that most rural counties lack even a single doctoral-level mental health professional and that only 3% of licensed psychiatrists practice in rural areas.

Men and women in the community that I serve are in need of treatment for dialysis three times per week and services for other illnesses. There is no mass transportation and many of these families have no transportation. It really can become a burden to the church community because the older adults must receive treatment. I believe that older African American women began suffering with dementia and Alzheimers because their bodies are breaking down and they cannot care for themselves. As a result it begins to work on their mental state.

Beliefs about mental illness, including stigmas related to mental illness, are prevalent in society whether or not an individual has direct experience with mental illness or not. Thus, beliefs have the potential to affect how an individual responds to symptoms of a mental illness in one's self or others. Does one seek care or not? Does one seek support or not? For this reason it is important to understand generally held beliefs about mental illness and to examine how these beliefs affect how individuals might cope with mental health problems. Examining beliefs in African Americans and stigma related to mental illness have found a long history of negativity. In an early study Silva de Crane and Spielberg found that African Americans perceived persons hospitalized for mental illness as different and inferior to normal people and believed these patients should be "restricted" to protect society. In the 1990s, a public opinion poll showed that 63 percent of African Americans believed depression was a personal weakness, and only 31 percent believed depression was a health problem (NMHA). This was a myth passed down from many generations and has caused a great deal of harm to African American women, including me. More recently, Thompson-Sanders et al., found that mental illness in the African American community was associated with shame and embarrassment and both the affected individual and the family had the illness.

I stopped crying when my children's names were mentioned when I declared in church while preaching a sermon that their deaths had caused me to have mental health issues. The day that I was able to acknowledge that I was mentally depressed out loud is the day that I stopped crying. I no longer cared what others thought, I did not care about stigma. I knew that I was suddenly set free. I am currently receiving psychological treatment because another traumatic experience that was crushing me. My current traumatic experience has forced me to seek counseling and through it I am examining my entire being since the loss of my family. I suffered in silence for many years.

Holistic understanding of psychiatric morbidity and service utilization is fostered by examination of individual- interpersonal and system-level factors. Factors at the individual level include client characteristics that predict service utilization and treatment outcomes. Individual-level factors have been the subject of considerable research and include race or ethnicity, religiosity, beliefs about mental health (i.e. stigma), and coping styles. At the interpersonal level, social support, stigma, and social distance influence willingness to initiate treatment and success in adhering to treatment recommendations. Social support in rural areas is central to the management of mental illness, in part because of limited access to specialty services, which is reflected in networks of informal care providers that are common in rural areas. Extended family, neighbors, and clergy often serve as alternatives to costly or inaccessible inpatient and outpatient services. The effectiveness of natural helpers in promoting positive change in mental health has been documented by several researchers. The Black church in particular has served a dominant role as an informal social service provider throughout its history) and its utility as an entry point for formal services has been the topic of considerable research. Studies suggest that churches still provide a wide range of preventive and treatment-oriented programs that contribute significantly to the psychological and physical well-being of their congregants. Services provided include substance abuse assistance as well as health screenings, education, and support. Churches in the community that I serve are compelled to serve. We believe that we are ordained by God to meet the needs of the poor. We believe that serving is the most significant part of our job. It does not matter whether it is HIV/AIDS awareness, substance abuse assistance, child care, GED training, single parenting, feeding the hungry, or clothing the naked, etc. We believe that it is our God-given duty to care for the "least of these." Yet, one of the most important areas in the lives of the African American community is underserved because we do not talk to our people about mental health treatment. We miss the boat when we see that our community is facing a mental health crisis. It is as though we do not see--do not experience the agony of the people who are suffering from mental depression, schizophrenia, and other mental health issues. We remind people that there is hope in Christ Jesus when it comes to salvation, but yet we fail to tell them that there can be hope for those who seek to be whole. Ezekiel was asked in Ezekiel 37, "can these bones live?" He said "Lord, you know." God said, "Prophesy to the bones," "prophesy to the breath.' "Come from the four winds, breathe. Breathe into these dead bones and let them live." The dry bones of African American women need a breath of life. They move through life carrying the burdens of their communities without a healing hand, without seeking to be made whole.

You will find the church and its members linked formally and informally in a system of care for the benefit of underserved or marginalized persons. We are linked informally through health fairs, health screenings, etc.

There are studies documenting the utility of lay persons, natural helpers, and especially religious leaders in the treatment of mental illness in a variety of settings. The focus on religious leaders has grown out of findings that paraprofessional counselors are often as effective as professionals in fostering positive change in recipients of services.

I wonder sometimes if God allowed me to go through the suffering that I endured so that I could help other women who are suffering. I wonder sometimes if God allowed me to turn the corner when I declared openly that I was mentally depressed. I wonder sometimes if God has allowed me to come to a place where I had to be totally dependent on him for my very existence. I wonder sometimes if I had to die in order to live so that I could tell women all over the world who find themselves in the midst of mental depression that there is a way back out of the dark hole. God leaves me to ponder these things as rebels often do. And even though I ponder and wonder out loud sometimes, I am filled with gratitude for what God has done in my life. I can see how God connected the dots for the me and the boys after their mom and their uncle's deaths, and how He kept on connecting the dots after my husband's death. I embrace the good and the bad events in my life for we have all fallen short. I know that every event in my life has brought me to this point by God's grace. I look at my past with a grateful heart, not with a heart filled with guilt and shame and not thinking about how I could have done things differently. I have found incredible power through the lens of my pain. Primarily, I am empowered to help the least of these. When I see the incredible things that "Heroes" are doing on CNN, I think to myself, the little bit that you are doing really is nothing. But I also realize that every little thing that you do in the lives of God's people helps to make a difference in their lives. They are grateful! I can see it in their eyes because I see things differently now that I have journeyed to the abyss and back. I see things from another perspective because my eyes are set on the kingdom of God.

I was reflecting a few days ago about not wanting to taste a mango that was offered to me by my mother-in-law many years ago. I refused to taste the mango because I saw it plucked from a tree, washed and the whole fruit lay on a plate on the dinner table. All I could think about was the thick looking skin on the fruit. My mother-in-law kept saying, "It is good, try it." I kept refusing. So she peeled the fruit when I was not looking, sliced it and put the slices in front of where I was to sit for dinner. The sweet aroma from the mango started to penetrate my nostrils and it got the best of me. I took my fork and gently took the smallest slice on the plate. I put the slice in my mouth and it was heavenly. I ate almost all of the fruit on the plate and several more mangoes from the tree; to the extent that the sides of my mouth were burned. That is how we are; we have images of something and if it does not meet with our approval we reject it. If it does not meet our cultural beliefs we reject it. We see individuals who have a mental illness and we reject that person because there is a stigma attached to people with mental illnesses. We want to alienate them, lock them up from society, because they are "acting crazy." We do not talk to the people or offer them help. So what does that say about those of us who are suffering from a mental illness? From society's perspective, we are not like them. We are different, we are stigmatized, and we are shunned. Is there any wonder that African American women like myself, turn to religion and refuse to seek the help that we so desperately need for our mental health?

With this writing, my life has been peeled back like a mango, to reveal a woman, who beneath the peeling demonstrates a kind of sweetness and resilience. Even though I was in a dark place for many years, I held on to the branch of life throughout the journey. My journey out of the abyss was nothing short of a miracle. I emerged to tell the story of God's sustaining power.

After I received my first appointment in June 2005, as the pastor of the United Methodist Church that I now serve, I really thought that Satan's attacks were over. I thought that I was in a safe place where I could minister to the people and continue to give my soul a rest. But that was not the case. I unwittingly stepped into hell's fire where the flames where flickering all around me; but by God's grace the flames did not touch me.

I shared how my mentor told me that I would never be a United Methodist and how she did everything that was within her power to stop me from transferring my credentials. She may have delayed the process but what she forgot was, while Satan may have some power, God has all power. If God sustained me through the devastation of losing all of my family in death, He would sustain me while she tried to kill my ministry. It has been difficult but He kept me. I am still standing in the United Methodist Church as a Methodist!

I had a dream about being in the middle of flames where everything was burning except me. Everything about that dream reminds me of a song that I love so much. It is entitled, "Through it All!" It goes something like this: "I've been through the fire and I've been through the storm; I've been broken into pieces, seen lightning flashing from above. But through it all I remembered that He loved me and He cared, and He will never put more on me than I can bear." When the flames started burning, I thought to myself, "With all the hell you've been through, this is nothing." God allowed the rebel to die so that she might live again!

REFERENCES

Alexander, Bryant, K. (2003). Fading, Twisting, and Weaving: An Interpretive Ethnography of the Black Barbershop As Cultural Space. *Qualitative Inquiry* 9: 105.

Areans, P.A & Reynolds, C.F. (2005). The impact of Psychosocial factors on late-life depression. *Bio Psychiatry* 58(4), 277-282.

Artinian, N.T., Washington, D.E., Flack, J.M., Hockman, E.M., & Jen, K.L. (2006). African American Women's Beliefs & Coping Behaviors. CDC, Atlanta, GA.

Avolio, B.J., Gardner, W.L., Walumbwa, F.O., Luthans, F., & May, D.R. (2004) Unlocking the Mask: A look at the process by which authentic leader's impact follower attitude and behaviors. *The Leadership Quarterly*, 15(6), 801-823

Baum, G. (1970). Man Becoming: God in Secular Experience. New York. Herder and Herder.

Begley, P. (2003). In pursuit of Authentic School Leadership Practices. In P. Begley and O. Johnson (Eds) *The Ethical Dynamics of School Leadership* (p 1-12). New York, New York. Kluwer Academic Press.

Beyer, P. (2010). Authentic Leadership in *extremis:* A study of Combat Leadership (Doctoral Dissertation) Retrieved November 22, 2014. ProQuest.

Boje, D. (1991). Consulting and change in the storytelling organization. *Journal of Organizational Change Management, 4, 7-17.*

Butler, J. (1988) Performative acts and gender constitution: An essay in phenomenology and feminist theory. *Theatre Journal.* 40(4), 519-531.

Chan, Hannah, & Gardner (2005). Authentic Leadership: Veritables In WL Gardner, BJ Avolio, & F.O. Walumbwa (Eds) A Leadership Theory and Practice: Origin, effects, & development. San Diego. Elsevier.

Conquergood, D. (2006). "Performance Ethnography: The Sage Handbook of Performance Studies. D. Soyini Madison & Judith Lamera (Eds.). Thousand Oaks. Sage Publication.

Cooper, C., Scandura, T., & Schriesheim, C. (2003). Challenges to developing authentic leadership theory and authentic leaders. *The Leadership Quarterly.* 16(3), 475-493.

Earl, Riggins. (1985). Dark Symbols Obscure Signs God, Self, and Community. Bloomburg Press.

Franklin, Robert. (1997). Another Day's Journey: Black Churches confronting the American Crisis in the slave mind. Augsburg Fortress.

Gardner & Schermehorn, (2004). Unleashing Performance Gain Through Positive Organizational Behavior and Authentic Leadership. *Organized Dynamics*. 33(3), 27-281.

Gardner, W.L., Avolio, B.J., Luthans, F., May, D.R., & Walumbwa, F. (2005). "Can you see the real me?" A self-based model of authentic leader and follower development. *The Leadership Quarterly, 16(3), 343-372.*

George (2003). Authentic Leadership: Re-creating the secrets of creating lasting value. San Francisco. Jossey-Bass.

George, Sim. McLean, & Mayer (2007). Discovering Your Authentic Leadership. *Harvard Business Review.* 85(2), 129-138.

Hughes, L.W. (2005) Spirit of Giving: *Relational transparency and humor in Authentic Leader-Follower relationships. In W.L. Gardner & BJ Avolio (Eds.) Authentic Leadership development: Monographs in Leadership and Management Series (Vol.3) Boston, MA. Elsevier. Jai Press.*

Ilies, R., Morgeson, F.P. & Nahrgang, J.D. (2005). Authentic leadership and eudaemonic well-being: Understanding leader-follower outcomes. *Leadership Quarterly, 16 373-394.*

Jackson, PR *(2004). Treatment of Anxiety and Depression Disorders in Patients with Cardiovascular Disease 325 (7445): 9339-943.*

Jones, D. (2000). Gender trouble in the workplace: 'Language and gender' meets 'feminist organizational communication.' In J. Holmes (Ed.).

Gendered Speech in Social Context*: Perspectives From gown and tows (pp.192-210)* Wellington, New Zealand: Victoria University Press.

Kernis, M.H. (2003). Target article: Toward a conceptualization of optimal self-esteem. *Psychological Inquiry, 14(1), 1-26.*

Klenke, K. (2005). The internal theater of the authentic leader: Integrating cognitive, affective, conative and spiritual facets of authentic leadership.

In W.L. Gardner, B.J. Avolio, & F.O. Walumbwa (Eds.). *Authentic leadership theory and practice: Origins, effects and development* (pp. 387-406). Oxford, UK: Elsevier Science.

Luthans, F., & Avolio, B.J. (2003). Authentic leadership development: A positive development approach: In K.S. Cameron. J.E. Morris, J.T (2010). The Impact of Authentic Leadership Behavior and Ethical Organizational Culture on Auditor Behavior.

(Doctoral Dissertation) Retrieved March 5, 2010 from www.sandiego.edu/leadership.

Musick, M.A. & D.R. Williams. (1998). The African American minister as a source of help for serious personal crisis: Bridge or barrier. Health, Education & Behavior 25(6), 759-943.

Olson, S. & R. Olson (2000). The "Xena" paradigm: Women's narratives of gender in the workplace. In J. Holmes (Ed.). Gendered speech in social context (pp. 178-191). Wellington, New Zealand: Victoria University Press.

Opatokun, Hasin & Hasan (2013). Authentic Leadership in Higher Learning Institutions: A Case Study of International Islamic University. International Journal of Leadership Studies. Malaysia.

Owen, C. (2003). The therapeutic alliance: The key to effective patient outcome? A descriptive review of the evidence in community mental health case management. 37(2), 169-183. *Australian & New Zealand Journal of Psychiatry*

Ready, D. (2002). How storytelling builds next generation Leaders. *MIT Sloan Management Review. 43(4), 63-69.*

Roux, S. (2010). The relationship between authentic leadership, optimism, self-efficacy and work engagement: An exploratory study (Doctoral Dissertation) Retrieved October 10, 2013 from https://scholar.sun.ac.za/bitstream/handle.10019.1/1/2182/Roux.%20S.M.pdf?sequence=1

Shamir, B., & Eilam, G. (2005) "What's your story?" A life- stories Approach to authentic leadership development. *The Leadership Quarterly, 16(3),* 395-417.

Sparrowe, R.T. (2005). Authentic leadership and thenarrative self. *The Leadership Quarterly*, 16(3), 419-439.

Thompson Sanders, V.L., Bazile. A., Akbar, M. (2004). African American's perceptions of psychotherapy and psychotherapists. *Professional Psychology Research & Experience.* 19-25.

Turner, V.W. (1986). Dewey, Dilthey, and drama: An essay in the anthropology of experience: In V.W. Turner and E.M. Bruner (Eds). *Anthropology of Experience* (pp.33-44) Urbana, Ill. University of Illinois.

Walumbwa, F.O., Avolio, B.J., Gardner, W.I., Wernsing, T.S., & Peterson, S.J. (2008). Authentic leadership: Development and validation of a theory based measure. *Journal of Management,* 34(1), 89.

Weedon, C. (1997). Feminist Practice and Post-structionalist Theory. (2nd Ed) Oxford, Blackwell.

West, C. & D. Zimmerman (1987). Doing Gender: *Gender and Society. 1(2), 125-151.*